Renew Yourself

Keys to Rejuvenation and Youthing

Dr. George Cromack, D.C., F.I.A.M.A.

Dedication

I dedicate this book to four outstanding teachers, each of whom has blazed a path and inspired countless people to greater levels of radiant health.

To **David Wolfe** — *for his ongoing contributions to Sunfood Nutrition ... and for thinking outside the box.*

◆ ◆ ◆

To **Gabriel Cousens, M.D.** — *for his contributions to the field of live food nutrition and for establishing the relationship between food and consciousness.*

◆ ◆ ◆

To **Dr. Norman Walker** — *for having lived his life as a remarkable example of what works and what's possible.*

◆ ◆ ◆

To **Peter Ragnar** — *for providing living proof of the existence of a fountain of youth.*

In their own way, each of these men has enriched my life and allowed me to serve humanity more fully.

---

*"**Nothing real can be threatened. Nothing unreal exists. Therein lies the peace of God."** - A Course in Miracles

Acknowledgments

To Lillian Müller for her inspirational book, "*Feel Great, Be Beautiful over 40: Inside Tips on How to Look Better, Be Healthier and Slow the Aging Process.*"

I would like to thank Laurie Masters of Precision Revision for her support and energy in editing and organizing the information in this book. She has been an invaluable aid in bringing my thoughts to clarity.

I would also like to thank Andrews Chuislekuda for his support in editing and helping to bring this book across the finish line.

I also wish to express my appreciation to Mom and Dad ... for providing the love, support, and space to finish this book.

Table of Contents

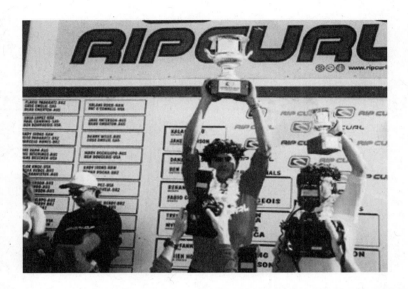

"*Dr. George Cromack has been monitoring my land-based training for the last few years. This included strength training, cardio, yoga, breathing exercises, deep relaxation and visualization, body-fat monitoring, supplements, and diet recommendations. He also played an integral role in my treatment and recovery from injuries. During the 2001 Rip Curl surfing semi-finals at Sunset Beach (Oahu, Hawaii) I was injured. Dr. George provided the treatment during the next hour that made it possible for me to compete in the finals and win!*"

— Myles Padaca, 2001 Vans Triple Crown champion

Introduction

Welcome to *Renew Yourself,* an easy-reference guide to creating your optimum state of well-being. This simple book consists of a brief, easy-to-read overview of several dozen tools that I have found to be most useful for healing both myself and my patients. In these pages, I have distilled a multitude of options down to just the ones I have found to produce the most predictable, dramatic results based upon my years of education, research and practice.

I chose to focus on practical application, rather than theory or philosophy. This book sticks to what works, why and how it works, the benefits you can expect, and how to do it. If you are feeling overwhelmed simply add a few topics that interest you to your daily routine. Try to practice the ideas you choose for 30 days straight, and see if you notice tangible results. As you feel better, it will be easier to continue. Every month try to integrate a new idea.

For additional help or guidance, I am available for phone consultation and coaching or you can visit my website www.RenewYourself.net. I also hold regular workshops where participants get to practice applying some of the tools while receiving personalized coaching.

In school, we don't receive an owner's manual that teaches us how to take care of our bodies. The world is filled with mixed and misleading messages. In *Renew Yourself,* you get the benefit of my insatiable curiosity and lifelong dedication to vibrant health.

May God guide you on your journey,

GEORGE CROMACK, D.C., F.I.A.M.A.

> *"Free will does not mean that you establish the curriculum, only that you can elect what you want to take at a given time."* - A Course in Miracles

PART 1 : DIET—CORE CONCEPTS

Live Foods for Health

An interesting ten-year study was conducted in the 1930s by Dr. Frances Pottenger. Approximately 900 cats were divided into two groups, one of which ate raw meat, and the other ate cooked meat. The raw food cats were able to reproduce healthy offspring for ongoing generations. Those fed cooked food bore many diseased or dead offspring, and the mothers eventually became sterile. Other negative physical and developmental issues in the cooked-food cats included degenerative and skin diseases, allergies, bone softening, skeletal deformities, and personality changes, including lethargy and aggressiveness.

These and other stunning differences between the cooked and raw food cats in Pottenger's study merely confirm the types of benefits I have observed among people who eat uncooked foods (myself included). As anyone who has taken a basic chemistry class can attest, heating a substance changes it ... and in the case of food, the changes are not positive, for humans or any other animals.

No other species of animal cooks its food, and for good reason — our digestive physiology was designed for foods in their natural form. Eating water-rich fruits and vegetables, unchanged from the way they occur in nature, is undoubtedly the most healthful dietary choice we can make.

According to Dr. Edward Howell, our enzyme supply is limited, and eating too much cooked food depletes our reserves. Temperatures above 118°F destroy the natural enzymes in food. You will read more on the importance of enzymes in Part 3.

Dr. Paul Kouchakoff demonstrated in the 1920s that "digestive leuko-cytosis" occurs when we eat cooked foods. This condition is an immune response in which white blood cells infiltrate the bloodstream, typically in response to infection, toxic chemicals, or trauma. In digestive leukocytosis, the white blood cells break down unusable compounds in these foods, which are devoid of the enzymes designed to help us digest them. Leukocytosis does not occur when we eat raw, unrefined, unprocessed foods.

I recommend that my patients strive to eat a diet of about 70–80% raw plant-based foods. Some people like to add cooked soups or steamed vegetables in the winter, although I would encourage you to instead try raw soups gently warmed in a Vita-Mix blender to a temperature of less than 118 degrees. Such soups are enzymatically alive and easy to digest (see the recipes in the "What to Eat" chapter). With its abundant fruits and warmer weather, summertime makes it easier to eat a raw diet. You might even experiment with eating all raw food for a month or two as a cleanse, and see what happens.

For More Information

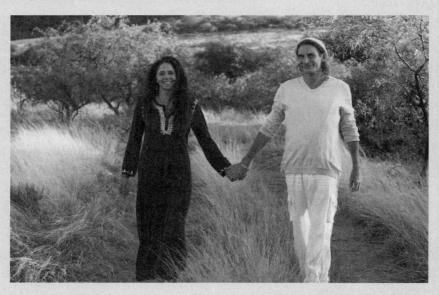

Dr. Gabriel Cousens' book *Conscious Eating*, offers a wealth of information for living a conscious and healthy life. At www.GabrielCousens.com, he offers a subscription-based video service that includes archives of his monthly three-hour Internet shows, with Q&A sessions at the end. Dr. Cousens is one of the most respected holistic medical doctors in the United States. He runs the Tree of Live Rejuvenation Center in Patagonia, Arizona (www.treeoflife.nu). A man of peace and extraordinary wisdom, Gabriel leads the field of live-food nutrition. His videos and books will change your life!

David Wolfe is one of the most energetic, fun, inspiring, and positive people

I have ever met. His book, *The Sunfood Diet Success System,* is a fabulous resource for new raw food enthusiasts. David is considered one of the world's top authorities on natural health, beauty nutrition, herbalism, chocolate, and organic superfoods. He holds a masters degree in living food nutrition and lectures internationally on the subject. He also hosts at least six health, fitness, and adventure retreats each year around the world. His books, lectures, events, and websites are a wealth of information about the living foods lifestyle. Check him out online at www.davidwolfe.com.

Matthew Monarch wrote a book called *Raw Spirit*, which I very much enjoyed. In a warm and friendly way, it relates Matt's journey from sickness to health, using raw foods and healthy lifestyle practices like the ones in this book. His second book, *Raw Success*, is also a great resource. Matt is committed to the raw lifestyle and passionate about spreading this message of health to others. His simple, accessible approach to going raw in a healthy and sustainable way are an inspiration to all.

Another inspiring story is that of Matt Monarch's beautiful wife, **Angela Stokes, who underwent a** remarkable transformation from a morbidly obese 21 year old weighing 294 lbs. to a healthy, vibrant 28-year old, at 138 lbs. Angela brings a unique brand of compassion and understanding to the raw food world, specializing in the emotional issues that underlie our eating choices. Her book *Raw Emotions,* is well worth a read if you struggle in any way with body weight/body image issues.

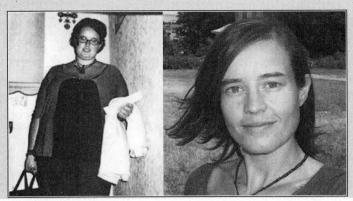

Shazzie, from the U.K., hC:\Users\AC\Documents\Projects\RenewYourself\Versions\shazzie.comas also written two excellent books, called *Detox Delight*, and *Detox Your World*. Her website, www.shazzie.com is famous for the humorous, inspiring online journal she wrote in 2000 as she transitioned to the raw food diet. Check out the articles at http://shazzie.com/life/articles/, particularly her 2009 piece called "The Raw Food Diet," a primer for the new raw food enthusiast that includes many useful links and resources. Shazzie's story, and her before & after pictures, are quite impressive! Surf her site, read her blog, and visit her wonderful online superstore. You will learn a great deal!

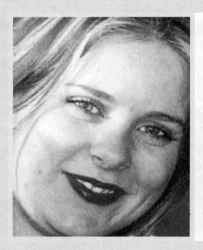 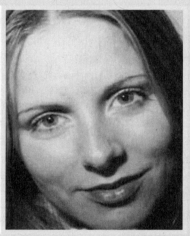

Len Foley is a prolific author, charismatic seminar facilitator, skilled interviewer, and one of the world's foremost creators of successful online communities. He hosts ongoing interviews with top leaders in the field of nutrition, health, and longevity, including David Wolfe, Gabriel Cousens, Peter Ragnar, and others. The interviews are archived online, along with many recorded David Wolfe lectures, at one of Len's "member sites," www.thebestdayever.com. Check them out.

Steve Prussack: Another excellent resource is Steve Prussack's weekly online Raw Vegan Radio show, at www.rawveganradio.com/wordpress/. This show, billed as "an audio encyclopedia on the living foods lifestyle," offers interviews with exciting guests in the field of health and raw food nutrition.

Understanding Body Type

> *"Diets need to take into consideration the time of year, your location, the weather, the type of work you do, whom you live with, your body type, and any imbalances you might have."*
>
> — Dr. George Cromack

Even though diet is a controversial and often emotionally charged issue, it is important to talk about it. The question is how big a difference can your diet make in how good you feels, and how quickly you heal? The answer is, HUGE! For guidance on dietary matters, I have come to appreciate the value of addressing the three basic constitutional body types—air, fire, and earth/water.

Air Type

These people are thin in spite of what they eat. They tend to move and think quickly and to be artistic, creative, and intelligent.

- When *balanced,* these people are mentally alert, have normal elimination, sleep soundly, have a strong immune function, and often feel a sense of exhilaration.
- When *imbalanced,* they exhibit dry skin, insomnia, fatigue, underweight, headaches, worry, difficulty with cold, and constipation.

Fire Type

This type of person tends to be of medium, muscular build, has lots of drive, and can be a little aggressive at times. People with red hair and fair, freckled skin are often strong fire types.

- When **balanced,** fire types have strong digestion, a sharp intellect, nice complexion, normal heat and thirst mechanisms, and feel content.
- When **imbalanced,** they experience rashes, heartburn, skin inflammation, irritability, excessive body heat, premature greying, and balding.

Earth/Water Type

These types of people tend to be heavy set and large boned. They move slowly and gain weight easily.

- When **balanced,** they often exhibit characteristics of strength, vitality, stamina, courage, generosity, and affection. They tend to have stable minds, strong immunity, and healthy joints.
- When **imbalanced,** earth/water types often experience oily skin, sinus congestion, overweight, slow digestion, allergies, mental dullness, and oversleeping.

When our bodies are in balance, things run smoothly. When they are out of balance, we suffer.

Each type correlates with a particular time of year. You can become severely upset if you partake in certain activities that aggravate your body type during that season. Thus, it is important to obtain a basic understanding of this model so you can realign yourself when things become unbalanced.

- June through September are fire months, and heat predominates. You want to avoid being in the mid-day sun, particularly if it is really hot where you are living and secondly you have a fire body type. Avoid eating hot foods with a fiery component during this time of year.
- Late September through the end of the year is air season, and the dry winds of autumn often prevail. If you have an air-type body, and you fly on a plane (which aggravates the air element) during the fall, you may experience an air type imbalance. To reset yourself, you would want to alter your diet toward an air-pacifying diet and activities.
- January through spring, earth/water season prevails. Have you ever

noticed how there are so many chesty, congested coughs and head colds during this time? A major sign of earth imbalance is phlegm. You need to eat a diet that pacifies congestion during these times.

Balancing Each Body Type

Now I will discuss how to balance the different body types. When balanced, the body is in homeostasis (a state of zero change) and experiences perfect health and rapid healing. Balancing involves counteracting imbalances with their opposite. So if the body is cold, this system recommends foods that are warming. It also uses the following six "tastes" to balance the body types.

- **Sweet:** milk, rice, pastas, sweets
- **Sour:** yogurt, cheese, lemon
- **Salty:** salt
- **Pungent:** ginger, hot peppers, cumin, and other sharp-tasting spices
- **Bitter:** green leafy vegetables, turmeric
- **Astringent:** lentils, beans

To rebalance the body types, eat more or less of the following tastes:

Fire—Increase: pungent, sour, salty **Decrease:** sweet, bitter, astringent
Air—Increase: pungent, bitter, astringent .. **Decrease:** sweet, sour, salty
Earth—Increase: sweet, sour, salty **Decrease:** pungent, bitter, astringent

Preventing Imbalances

Air

- Eat and sleep at regular times.
- Stay warm in cold weather.
- Drink plenty of warm liquids, including soups, broths, and herbal teas.
- Avoid stimulants.

- Use some Himalayan Crystal Salt with your foods.
- Oils pacify an air imbalance, so adding krill, coconut, hemp seed, or other oils to your soups and smoothies is beneficial.
- Giving yourself an abhyanga warm sesame oil head and foot massage (see page 132) is excellent, especially before bed.

Fire

- Keep cool in hot weather and exercise in moderation.
- Avoid alcohol, smoking, excessive heat and sun exposure, stress, spicy, sour, and salty food, and coffee.
- Eating watermelon, or drinking celery juice with young coconut water, are excellent cooling choices for hydrating yourself during the summer.

I don't suggest eating a South African watermelon in the U.K. in January. This creates imbalance, as you are already wet and cold, because it is earth/water season. Eating watermelon will cool you down further in the cold season, regardless of your body type.

Earth/Water

- Avoid excessive rest and oversleeping.
- Get plenty of exercise.
- Don't overeat heavy, oily foods.
- Stay warm in cold weather.
- Favor spicy, bitter, and astringent tasting foods.
- Avoid dairy products.
- Drink ginger tea.

Having a cold is an earth/water imbalance. Eating dairy products during this time slows recovery, as dairy products are mucus forming.

For More Information

Conscious Eating: Dr. Gabriel Cousens' excellent book will teach you how to tailor a 70–80% live food diet according to your body type, for health and longevity. You can get a copy at www.RenewYourself.net by clicking on the Books section.

Digestion

Proper digestion results in efficient assimilation of nutrients, which fortify the body and ultimately become the essential nerve energy of the body. When this life force is in plentiful supply, we have good health and strong immune function. When it is deficient, we become weak, tired, and diseased.

This energy is produced at every stage of digestion, so taking steps to ensure good digestion is a vital part of creating health. Improper digestion produces metabolic waste products and erodes health. It is imperative that you develop the following habits, to increase your digestive fire and metabolic efficiency.

- Upon arising, drink a glass of warm water with a dash of lemon juice and raw honey.
- Make lunch the largest meal of the day.
- Avoid eating after 6:30 in the evening.
- Sip half a cup of plain hot water from a thermos every hour throughout the day. You may add a pinch of fresh ginger or turmeric, or a few fennel seeds. During the summer, use room-temperature water instead.
- Avoid eating reheated and leftover food.
- Avoid cold beverages, especially ice-cold water.
- Eat to about ¾ of your capacity or until you feel satisfied but light.
- Eat at the same time each day.
- Avoid eating before the previous meal is digested.
- Do not heat honey in any way.
- Consider fasting one day a week on warm water.
- Take a few capsules of Triphala (see page 53) before bed.
- Eat an abundance of fresh, organically grown food.
- Eat your food in a peaceful environment, and spend several minutes in silence after completing each meal.
- Chew your food thoroughly.
- Supplement with hydrochloric acid (available from a health-food store) and enzymes (see page 59) if you are over 50 or experience digestive difficulty.

- Use the appropriate churnas (spice blends) for your body type (see "For More Information," below).
- Take a capsule or two of the appropriate herbal digestive aid for your body type (see "For More Information," below).

For More Information

Digestive aids for your body type: If you are an air body type, choose *Herbal Di-Gest* for relief of gas and bloating. Pittas should choose *Aci-Balance* for acid reflux and heartburn. And earth/water body types should take *MA154 Digest Plus* for slow digestion.

Churnas: These spice blends are custom formulated for each body type, to support digestive health and optimum nutrition. These items are also available upon request through my website.

All of the above items are available upon request. Please visit www.RenewYourself.net and click Contact. I will get back to you promptly.

Managing Blood Sugar

There is a lot of talk in the world of health and nutrition about the glycemic index (GI), a chart that measures how quickly the carbohydrates you eat turn to sugar in your blood. But there is a related index, called "glycemic load" (GL), which tells you how much of that carbohydrate is in a serving of a particular food. Glycemic load is the better predictor of how much a food raises blood sugar, but both concepts are important to understand if you wish to keep your blood sugar levels in a healthy range.

Any time you eat carbohydrate-rich foods, glucose enters your bloodstream. If you are eating healthy unprocessed whole foods, and your body is functioning correctly, this is not a problem. The sugar quickly leaves the bloodstream and, with the help of insulin, is deposited into the cells of your body, where it serves as fuel.

However, some foods interfere with insulin function, causing sugar to pile up and have a hard time exiting the bloodstream. When this occurs, your cells become starved for energy. And if it happens repeatedly for long periods of time, you can end up with damage to the nerves, eyes, kidneys, hearts, and blood vessels (for starters).

High GL foods cause spikes in insulin. If insulin levels stay chronically high, our insulin receptors become desensitized over time, then the pancreas has to secrete more insulin to do the same job. This is a dangerous condition that leads to blood sugar instability and eventually diabetes and other blood sugar metabolic disorders. Increased insulin also causes health problems such as the following:

- Increased fat storage
- Decrease in human growth hormone
- Increase in cortisol (the "stress hormone")
- Decrease in testosterone
- Decrease in DHEA
- Adrenal fatigue
- Mood swings

- Decreased immune function
- Increased inflammation

Examples of foods with a low glycemic load are vegetables, seeds, nuts, and berries. High GL foods include corn flakes, pastries, pastas, mashed potatoes, candies, crackers, pancakes, and rice. Many of the starches contain "opioid" (opium-like) substances that make them somewhat addictive. Refined sugars stimulate beta endorphin receptors in the brain, creating addictive cravings as well. Your body interprets high sugar levels as stress and increases insulin. This is just one more reason to eliminate refined, processed, carbohydrate foods from your diet.

Fresh fruits are another story. You may be surprised to learn that most fruits rank either low or medium on the GI, and low on the GL. Only watermelon is (barely) high on the glycemic index, but it has a low glycemic load (see table on the next page). If you eat *whole* fruit with the fiber intact, you will find the blood sugar issues are not a problem, as long as you keep your dietary fat low to moderate and use healthy fats. High levels of fat in the diet interfere with insulin's ability to do its work.

I encourage you to scroll through the GI/GL table listed in the "For More Information" section below, to familiarize yourself with the types of foods that tend to spike insulin and blood sugar. Or if you want to keep things simple, just stick to whole, fresh, unprocessed, plant foods. Your body will thank you.

Food	Glycemic Index (GI) Low 1-55	Med 56-69	High 70+	Glycemic Load (GL) Low 1-10	Med 11-19	High 20+
RAW FOODS						
Strawberries	40 (low)			1 (low)		
Watermelon	72 (high)			4 (low)		
Peaches	42 (low)			5 (low)		
Apples	38 (low)			6 (low)		
Pineapples	59 (med)			7 (low)		
Grapes	46 (low)			8 (low)		
Bananas	52 (low)			12 (med)		
Carrots	47 (low)			3 (low)		
Beets	64 (med)			5 (low)		
COOKED FOODS						
Bran cereal	42 (low)			8 (low)		
Popcorn	72 (high)			8 (low)		
Corn, sweet	54 (high)			9 (low)		
Whole wheat bread	71 (high)			9 (low)		
Wild rice	57 (med)			18 (med)		
Spaghetti	42 (low)			20 (high)		
White rice	64 (med)			23 (high)		
Baked potatoes	85 (high)			26 (high)		
Sweet potatoes	61 (med)			17 (med)		

Source: www.mendosa.com/common_foods.htm

For More Information

Glycemic index and glycemic load: Comprehensive information about both glycemic index and glycemic load are available online at this website: www.mendosa.com/gilists.htm, including tables with GI and GL data for 750 foods.

Acid/Alkaline Balance

The pH scale, which ranges from 0 to 14, measures the acidity or basicity (alkalinity) of a solution. Pure water has a neutral pH (neither acidic nor basic) of 7.0. A pH of less than 7 means the solution is acidic. A pH of more than 7 means the solution is basic. A lower pH is more acidic; a higher pH is more basic.

You can use inexpensive drugstore litmus paper to test the pH of your saliva and/or urine (see "For More Information" for a link to a detailed procedure). The pH of your urine after you eat or drink indicates your level of alkaline mineral reserves, and how well your body is able to handle the acid residues left behind by those foods and drinks.

Both your urinary and saliva pH should be approximately neutral, ranging about 6.8 to 7.2. If your pH is lower than 6.8, your body is overly acidic. This creates an environment that is said to be more conducive to viruses and tumors. It also decreases your energy potential.

If you are acidic, you can increase your alkalinity by adding more fresh fruits and vegetables to your diet and reducing the amount of meat, starches, refined sugars, and carbonated soda you consume. One can of soda is so acidic that it takes 30 glasses of extremely alkaline water (pH 10—only available from special alkaline water machines) to neutralize it!

Excess acids are often stored in the tissues and joints, and they will exit via the organs of elimination during cleansing. So don't be surprised if your pH becomes temporarily more acidic as you clean up your diet.

During this transition time, it is important to drink freshly juiced green drinks, E3Live® Aquabotanical (see page 37) and Pure Synergy superfood (see page 47). Incorporating fresh green juice drinks is the quickest way I know to start increasing your alkaline reserves.

What to Eat

While no one diet is perfect for all people, at all times, in all locations, general principles can be applied to a wide audience. Let's begin with the core foods.

A healthful diet should be rich in vital nutrients, including enzymes, fiber, vitamins, minerals, antioxidants, phytochemicals, and long-chain omega-3 fatty acids. It should consist primarily of alkaline-forming plant foods that are easy to digest and that rank low to medium on the glycemic index (see page 13).

I recommend making an effort to buy your food fresh and in season from a farmers' market, selecting organically grown produce whenever possible. The food should not only look good but should taste great. Organically grown food is more nutrient dense and eliminates the toxic effects of pesticides, commercial fertilizers, and genetic modification. Buying commercial produce out of season, from thousands of miles away, usually results in expensive, nutritionally inferior food that has less flavor than fresh food in season.

The basis for a healthy diet is an abundance of fresh, colorful whole and juiced fruits, vegetables, and sprouts, as well as wheatgrass, and healthy fats and proteins from nuts, seeds, avocados, and olives. Strive to incorporate all the colors of the rainbow in your weekly array of fruits and vegetables. Eating highly pigmented foods increases immunity, mental clarity, and speed of healing from disease or pain. It is also said to enhance energy, flexibility, contentment, and skin clarity.

There are much better alternatives to the well advertised and highly marketed commercial man-made synthetic vitamins that recent research is proving have little to no benefit and in some cases even create harm. There is a real benefit to supplementation with superfoods and whole-food concentrates derived from the healthiest nutrient dense, prana-rich live food possible. I am convinced that supplementing our diet with an abundance of these foods extends and enhances our lives. They are essential for increasing our capacity to handle the barrage of dietary and environmental toxins we face each day, and for helping us to function at an optimal level of health and happiness.

A Transition Plan

To begin incorporating the foods and supplements in parts 2 & 3 of this book, I suggest two initial steps: (1) follow the "Smoothie Recipe and E3Live® Instructions" on page 42, and (2) start introducing a salad or blended soup (like the ones described under "Basic Recipes" on page 20) into your daily routine. After a few weeks, adding a freshly juiced green vegetable drink to your day, about 30 to 60 minutes before dinner. Then in a few more weeks, introduce some Pure Synergy (see page 47) to your morning smoothies and a little to your afternoon juice.

E3Live® and Pure Synergy can help fill in many nutritional deficits, and they have a major stabilizing effect on blood sugar levels. When blood sugar is stable and nutritional needs are met, most cravings for junk food disappear.

When your transition is complete, your daily regimen might look something like the following:

- Super smoothie for breakfast (see page 21).
- Fruit or vegetable salad and/or warmed blended veggie soup for lunch.
- Fresh vegetable juice in the late afternoon.
- A large salad with a healthy entrée for dinner.

As you cleanse your body, you become more conscious and open to learning. And your concept of what constitutes a healthy meal changes over time. By eating lots of nutrient-dense superfoods during the day, and starting dinner with a freshly made green drink, you will find that your blood sugar level remains stable. As a result, you will experience fewer cravings for heavier and undesirable foods at dinnertime, and you will also require smaller quantities of food.

Foods to Avoid

You should avoid commercial produce, processed foods (most packaged multi-ingredient foods), refined sugars and flours, saturated fats, trans fatty acids (anything that contains "hydrogenated" or "partially hydrogenated" oils), genetically modified food, and impure water. These items lead to low energy, depression, frequent colds, skin problems, slow recovery from illness or injury, chronic pain, irritability, increased medical bills, and premature aging.

Meat, fish, and dairy are dangerously high in protein and fat, raise cholesterol, contain no fiber, can contain growth hormones, antibiotics, as well as concentrations of concentrate environmental toxins and pesticides. Research from the Max Planck Institute shows cooking of animal foods causes protein coagulation, decreasing assimilation by 50%.

Commercial breakfast cereals, donuts, and other pastries are high on the glycemic index and lead to insulin surges. They are difficult to digest, devoid of nutrients, and filled with chemicals and additives. Potato chips and other fried foods are equally devastating to the health and also contain carcinogenic trans fatty acids.

Having lived in Europe, I realized that most Europeans are much more aware of the dangers of genetically modified (GM) foods than Americans are. In Europe, these foods are known as "frankenfoods." In the U.S., they appear indirectly in many foods and do not require labeling. It is estimated that three-quarters of the foods in U.S. supermarkets contain genetically modified organisms (GMOs), including any foods with nonorganic soy or corn, as well as tomatoes, potatoes, sweet corn, rice, and products made with rapeseed (canola oil) and sugarcane. In spite of what Monsanto and its lobbyist try to tell you, GM food is not safe. Nobel prize-winning scientists have refused large sums of money to endorse GM foods.

Make no mistake: GMOs are bad news. Educate yourself on the topic, and avoid them to the greatest extent possible.

Basic Recipes

I'll wrap up this chapter with five simple recipes. Many of the ingredients that may be unfamiliar to you will be discussed in Part 3, "Diet — Superfoods & Supplements."

1. Fruit Salad
- 1 cup organic berries
- 1 apple, chopped
- 1 peach, chopped
- ½ cup goji berries
- ½ cup raw seeds or nuts

Soak the seeds or nuts for 8 hours in clean water and drain. Blend with 1/3 cup water. Then add about ¼ teaspoon each of cinnamon, nutmeg, and ginger, 1 teaspoon of monuka honey, and ¼ teaspoon Himalayan Crystal Salt, and continue to blend. Pour the sauce over the fruit salad.

I recommend soaking seeds and nuts because they contain *phytates* — enzyme inhibitors that keep the seed or nut from sprouting until sufficient water is available. Phytates also inhibit digestion. Soaking off the phytates and blending the seeds or nuts makes them easier to digest.

2. Basic Vegetable Salad
- 1 cup organic spinach leaves, washed and chopped
- 1 to 2 cups mixed salad greens
- 1 celery stalk, chopped
- ½ small yellow pepper, chopped
- ½ cup pitted olives or avocado
- ½ cup hijiki seaweed, soaked
- ¼ cup slivered almonds or pumpkin seeds, soaked

3. Salad Dressing or Veggie Dip

Blend the following:

- 1/3 cup sesame tahini or blended soaked sunflower seeds
- ½ cup water
- 1 teaspoon freshly squeezed lemon juice
- 1 teaspoon manuka honey
- ½ teaspoon Himalayan Crystal Salt
- 3 sun-dried tomato slices
- ¼ teaspoon ginger

4. Blended Veggie Soup

Blend the following, and slowly warm to about 110 degrees:

- 1 cup spinach
- 1 cup celery
- ½ sweet bell pepper
- ½ cucumber
- 6 sun-dried tomato slices
- 1 teaspoon hemp seed oil
- 1 teaspoon freshly squeezed lemon juice
- ¾ teaspoon Himalayan Crystal Salt
- 1 teaspoon manuka honey
- 1½ cups water
- ¼ cup almonds or sunflower seeds, soaked
- ½ teaspoon fresh ginger
- 1 tablespoon dulse flakes
- ¼ cup avocado

5. Dr. George's Super Smoothie

Blend all of the following:

- 8 oz. freshly squeezed apple or orange juice
- ½ cup frozen organic berries (or if not available, frozen banana)
- 2 tablespoons E3Live®
- 1 teaspoon raw coconut oil

- 1 tablespoon organic hemp oil
- 1 teaspoon organic bee pollen
- ½ teaspoon raw royal jelly
- 1 teaspoon raw manuka honey
- 1 teaspoon E3Live® BrainON®
- 1 tablespoon Pure Synergy powder
- ¼ teaspoon Himalayan Crystal Salt
- 1 teaspoon Pure Radiance C
  (available at www.RenewYourself.net, under the Pure Synergy tab.)

This last recipe is a very potent, easy-to-digest super tonic smoothie that tastes great! It is important to take it first thing in the morning on an empty stomach and not to eat anything else for at least 25 minutes. This allows the nutrients to get into your bloodstream. This blend is extremely balancing to the blood sugar, so it tends to decrease hunger binges resulting from low blood sugar. Start slowly, and if you are transitioning from a heavy traditional diet, decrease the quantity of all ingredients by half.

Optimally you should already be following my instructions for letting your body adapt to E3Live® (see page 37) for at least 30 days before trying this super smoothie. Its alchemical combination will have your endorphin centers pumping, taking you toward experiences of heightened well-being and natural euphoria. This all happens in a healthy, balanced way, while your body becomes stronger each day.

For More Information

Honest Food Guide: I recommend downloading a free copy of Mike Adams's Honest Food Guide at www.honestfoodguide.org. Try eating less of the foods on the left (disease) side and more of the foods on the right (health) side.

PART 2: DIET—FRESH PLANT FOODS

Leafy Greens

Chlorophyll is the life blood of the plant. It is sun energy. It is light energy. By taking in chlorophyll-rich dark-green leafy vegetables, we dispel the darkness inside and regenerate our blood.

The chlorophyll molecule is almost identical to the hemoglobin molecule in our blood cells, except that hemoglobin has iron in the center, and chlorophyll has magnesium in the center.

PLANT CHLOROPHYLL
MAGNESIUM AT THE CENTER

HUMAN BLOOD HEMOGLOBIN
IRON AT THE CENTER

Calorie for calorie, leafy greens may be the most concentrated source of nutrients we can eat. In addition to life-giving chlorophyll, greens are a rich source of vitamins, (including A, C, E, K, and many of the B vitamins), minerals (including iron, calcium, potassium, folate, zinc, manganese, and magnesium), enzymes, phytonutrients, antioxidants, and the soft, soluble fiber humans need for optimal digestion. They even contain small but adequate amounts of essential omega-3 fatty acids and essential amino acids.

Often when I ask patients about their intake of greens I get a puzzled look, or they say that they don't like greens. Occasionally someone proudly mentions that he or she eats a salad with dinner every day. This usually means a dinner salad made with commercially grown iceberg lettuce, some carrots, and cucumber with bottled salad dressing.

Sorry, this isn't going to cut it. The standard American diet is a recipe for a severely demineralized person. In fact, ninety-nine percent of the population is drowning in acid and lacking in alkaline minerals like calcium, potassium, magnesium, and sodium. When you eat acid-forming foods (coffee, refined sweets, pastries, meat, dairy, pasta, flour products, colas, etc.) your body constantly draws on alkaline mineral reserves from your bones, in an attempt to buffer the acidic diet.

Drinking milk in an attempt to obtain calcium won't help the situation. In fact, the countries with the highest dairy consumption have the highest rate of osteoporosis. The Scandinavian countries are a perfect example.

Instead, you need to eat lots of green leafy vegetables to remineralize your body. And as you move to a cleaner diet, you will need even more greens than usual, because the volume of toxins being eliminated requires extra alkaline minerals to neutralize them as they travel through the bloodstream on their way out.

I encourage you to rethink the way you eat greens, elevating them in status from small side salads to generous -sized entrées, every night of the week. And be sure to take in plenty of additional greens in the form of freshly juiced green vegetable drinks, sunflower and alfalfa sprout juices, wild greens foraged in nature, wheatgrass juice, and generous doses of the green supplements and superfoods described in Part 3, particularly E3Live®. At the same time, avoiding acidifying, demineralized foods is vital.

For More Information

You can find excellent information to help you incorporate leafy green vegetables into your diet in the books mentioned at the end of the Live Foods chapter.

Wild edibles: You might also consider reading up on wild foods, or taking a wild food foraging class. Here is a wonderful website for the wild food enthusiast:http://wildfoodplants.com/resources.

Fruit and Vegetable Juices

Juicing can be a powerful tool in healing and rejuvenating your body. One of the most notable proponents of juicing was Dr. Norman Walker, who is said to have lived to age 116, in good health until the end. Interestingly enough, he was in relatively poor health in his 60s, until he took up a diet of mostly raw fruits, vegetables, and seeds with plenty of freshly squeezed vegetable juices.

Why is juicing so important? Because all of us are seriously demineralized! Most of us from have grown up on a conventional diet of processed, chemically treated food. The mainstream diet generally includes only small amounts of commercially grown produce, and lots of meat, dairy, refined sugar, and starches. These foods are very low in minerals and are acid forming. This means they draw on your alkaline mineral reserves to buffer their acidity. This type of a diet is a major contributing factor in osteoporosis.

Juicing is an excellent way to start replenishing your body with easy-to-assimilate organic minerals. These minerals also help to smooth out the de-toxification process that often accompanies improvements in diet and lifestyle.

By stripping away the pulp, we can extract juice from a much larger quantity of produce than we would be able to eat. Vegetable fiber can be difficult to digest in large quantities. Freshly squeezed juices make it possible to use juices therapeutically. Drinking 20 oz. a day of a green juice blend will do wonders for your health.

Although the possibilities are endless, here is a simple juice recipe I like: juice celery, cucumber, kale, apple, and a small amount of ginger with a squeeze of lemon and a pinch of sea salt.

Choosing a Juicer

After a lot of research and experimentation, I chose to sell a small number of excellent juicers on my website. Here is a brief description of each, to help you decide on the best model for your needs.

The **Champion** juicer processes all fruits easily and does a pretty good job on green leafy vegetables such as spinach and kale, but it will not juice wheatgrass. I have owned a Champion juicer for more than 15 years, and they are powerful and dependable, with a motor that lasts a very long time. I find them quick and easy to clean—I can clean mine in 3 to 4 minutes.

I have also owned a **Green Star** juicer, which uses a magnetized double-auger blade that spins at a slow speed. This model is more efficient at juicing green leafy vegetables, and it will also juice wheatgrass. The juice keeps a little longer, as it oxidizes less due to the magnets and the slower movement of the double-auger blades. The Green Star costs about $175 more than the Champion and takes significantly longer to clean, but if you plan to juice a lot of green leafy vegetable, it's well worth the investment.

The **Omega** and **Solo Star** are single-auger juicers that offer a compromise between the Champion and the Green Star. Both juice greens a bit more efficiently than the Champion but are a little slower at juicing fruits. They offer less oxidation, cost less than the Green Star, and are quicker to clean.

At this stage of the game, I am happy with my Champion juicer, as it is a little less efficient, but much quicker to do the juicing and the cleanup.

For More Information

Juicers: The four juicers described above are available on my website. Visit www.RenewYourself.net and click the Appliances section.

Juicing books by Dr. Norman Walker: I highly recommend reading Dr. Walker's three juicing books: *Become Younger*, *Fresh Vegetable and Fruit Juices*, and *The Natural Way to Vibrant Health*. You can find these books under the Books section at www.RenewYourself.net.

Wheatgrass Juice

Wheatgrass is the young grass shoots of the wheatberry, about a week of age. It must be juiced for humans to digest it. Wheatgrass is extremely nutrient dense and particularly rich in chlorophyll and enzyme content, making it highly cleansing and rejuvenating. It is essentially liquid sunshine and contains an incredible amount of light energy.

When grown indoors in trays and then squeezed into juice, wheatgrass provides a myriad of health benefits. Here are some highlights:

- One shot has the nutritional value of 2 lbs. of green vegetables
- Absorbs 92 of the known 102 minerals from the soil
- Alkalizes the body
- Detoxifies cellular fluids
- Boosts immunity, fights infection, heals wounds
- Improves digestion and promotes regularity
- Chelates out heavy metals
- Purges the liver
- Purifies the bloodstream and increases its oxygen- and nutrient-carrying capacity
- Improves skin and hair
- Energizes the body and mind
- Helps balance blood sugar levels and normalize blood pressure

I recommend starting with one shot of wheatgrass a day in the morning, on an empty stomach. This should be followed by a large glass of warm clean water. Then allow 20 minutes before eating anything. If you eat a lighter diet, you can also drink some wheatgrass juice mid-afternoon. After taking a shot a day for a month you can experiment with taking two shots a day.

Growing Wheatgrass

The nice thing about growing your own wheatgrass for juicing is that it is very inexpensive and tastes much fresher than store-bought juice made 8 to 48 hours earlier. Wheatgrass juice is much smoother when it is grown on nutrient-dense soil from organic seed, and supplemented with liquid kelp and seawater. One cup of soaked seed will yield one tray of wheatgrass, which makes about 6 to 8 ounces of juice. So if you are going to do one shot a day, you need to plant one tray every six days.

Soak one cup of wheatberries for 4 hours (in hot weather) to 12 hours (in cold weather), at room temperature. For easy rinsing, use a clean, wide-mouthed canning jar with a screened sprouting lid, or cover with a porous cloth secured with a rubber band. Drain and rinse, then place the jar at an angle so it can drain. When the seeds get little white sprouts, they are ready to plant.

Buy a half dozen 6×12" planting trays and some organic potting soil. Line the tray with a large plastic garbage bag. Spread about 1½ inches of dampened soil over the tray. Pour the seed onto the tray and spread it so that the seeds form a thick, solid single layer. Water generously and fold the plastic bag over the top of the tray to cover the wheatgrass.

Spray the wheat sprouts about twice a day with a dilute solution of sea water and liquid kelp. After two days, you can pull back the cover. Continue to water once a day and mist twice a day with the solution. Put the tray in a well-ventilated area that has indirect sunlight. When the grass is about six inches high, it is ready to start harvesting. Cut it with a knife or scissors. You will need a special wheatgrass juicer, either manual or electric.

Try it for 30 days and you will notice a nice health improvement.

For More Information

Z Star wheatgrass juicer: I recommend the Z Star Manual Juicer from Tribest, an extremely efficient single-auger machine that extracts the maximum juice from every blade of wheatgrass. Since it doesn't require electricity, you can use it when you travel, so you never have to miss a day of wheatgrass. Available at www.RenewYourself.net under Appliances.

Sprouts

Sprouts are the embryonic form of plants that are edible at their first stage of life. They are an amazing nutrient-rich living food. Nature supercompacts seeds with the energy necessary to perform the miracle of growth as the seed begins its transformation into a plant. You can be a personal witness to and beneficiary of this process right in your kitchen.

Sunflower Greens

Sunflower greens are baby sunflower plants—the young sprouts grown from unhulled (whole) sunflower seeds when they split apart into the first two leaves, called cotyledons. (They should not be confused with sunflower *sprouts,* which are sunflower seeds with their hulls removed that are soaked then sprouted for a day or two until a tail emerges.)

Sunflower greens are loaded with chlorophyll, enzymes, vitamins, minerals, amino acids, and other nutrients. They are a rich source of lecithin, which helps with breakdown and digestion of fats. They are quite crunchy and flavorful in salads, and are excellent and tasty juiced.

Grow sunflower greens in soil, using the method described for wheatgrass. You can also grow a variety of other baby greens in this manner, including cabbage, radish, arugula, buckwheat "lettuce," and pea "shoots." Feel free to add them generously to your diet. I recommend that you also juice a quarter cup's worth of baby sunflower greens several times a week and add it to your afternoon green vegetable drink.

Sprouts Grown in Jars or Bags

Sprouting in bags or jars is an inexpensive, tasty way to add high-enzyme, nutrient-dense food to your diet. It is also an easier undertaking than growing baby greens in soil, so you might want to try this method first when dipping your toe into the world of sprouting. I recommend starting to experiment with alfalfa seeds, as they are easy to sprout and familiar to most people.

After you get the hang of sprouting alfalfa, you can expand your repertoire include a wide variety of nutrition-packed sprouts, including grains (wheat, barley, rye, kamut, quinoa, etc.), beans (mung, lentil, garbanzo, adzuki, etc.), greens (alfalfa, broccoli, radish, onion, cabbage, kale, turnip, clover, cress, arugula, etc.), and many others. The bag method is better for sprouting tiny seeds (like amaranth) and large beans, and it can even be used for gelatinous seeds like chia and flax.

You can use sprouts grown in this manner the same way you eat soil-grown baby greens—either in salads or other raw entrees, or juiced and consumed as shots or as part of your afternoon vegetable juice.

Sprouting in Jars

Place 1 or 2 tablespoons of sprout seeds in a wide-mouthed glass canning jar. If you don't have a special screened sprouting lid, cover the jar with cheese-cloth or mesh, and secure it with a rubber band. Wash, swirl and drain the seeds. Then add a cup of water and soak for 4–8 hours. Drain the water, then rinse and drain again with fresh water. Invert the jar and set it in an angled dish drainer or prop it in a bowl or sink at a 45-degree angle to drain. Avoid sprouting in direct sunlight. Refill the jar with water, rinse, and drain 2–3 times a day, always keeping it angled for proper drainage.

Sprouting times range from 12 hours (quinoa) to one week (various), depending on the type of seed. When the sprouts have leaves, move the jars to a window with indirect sunlight for the last day or two, so the sprouts can develop chlorophyll and begin to green.

When you are ready to harvest, rinse your sprouts well, and wash off as many hulls as possible. Eat your sprouts immediately, or store them in the refrigerator for up to one week.

Sprouting in bags

According to "Sproutman" Steve Meyerowitz, sprouting in bags is a superior alternative to the jar method. In his words, "jars were never designed for sprouting. Their popularity has more to do with their wide availability and free cost than with their merits as a gardening tool."

Some of the advantages of bag sprouting include:
- All sprouts get air (jars have relatively poor air circulation).
- 100% drainage (tilted jars don't drain fully and can harbor mold).
- Can expand & contract according to volume (jars are fixed size).
- Lightweight and easily portable for traveling, camping, boating (jars are breakable, heavy, and cumbersome to travel with).
- Saves space (bags hang from a hook or knob to save precious counter or refrigerator space).
- Just "dip and hang" (four-step jar sprouting takes more time).

Give bag sprouting a try ... I think you will love it!

For More Information

Sprouting information: For more great information, including guidelines on soaking and sprouting times, read "A Brief Overview on How to Sprout," at http://chetday.com/sprouts.html.

Sunflower greens: Visit this website for helpful growing information: http://www.rawfoods-livingfoods.com/sunflower-sprouts.html.

3-Jar Super Sampler Seed Sprouting Jar Kit: Handy Pantry Sprouting offers a complete starter kit, which includes three jars, an instruction book, and ten 4-oz. bags of seeds. Get yours at www.handypantry.com/product/3JSK.

Sproutman's 100% Natural Hemp Sprout Bag: You can find many sprout bag products online. The Sproutman's version is a good one. You can get if from www.sproutman.com/sprouters/sproutmans-natural-hemp-sprout-bag.
Be sure to watch the two-minute sprout bag demonstration video.

Click on Books at www.RenewYourself.net for more books on sprouting.

PART 3: DIET—
SUPERFOODS &
SUPPLEMENTS

E3Live® Aquabotanical

> **"Supplementing your diet with E3Live® immediately is one of the fastest ways I know of to kick start your return to optimum health."**
>
> — Dr. George Cromack

The term "superfood" has now entered our mainstream culture. In general, the term refers to a single food with a diverse nutrient profile that offers substantial health benefits for your body, your mind and, in the rarest of cases, your emotions.

Some consider seaweeds like hijiki, wakame, arame, and dulse, and the seaweed extract fucoidan, to be superfoods. These products are rich in trace minerals and capable of flushing toxins out of the body. Goji berries, bee pollen, royal jelly, maca, aloe vera, wheatgrass, spirulina, and chlorella, among others, are also considered superfoods.

True superfoods are dense in vitamins, minerals, antioxidants, and other nutrients, and they are fresh and alive with enzymatic action, making them easy to digest. They generally impart a direct physical sense of enhanced energy, and many also stimulate subtle energy channels to increase the circulation of life-force energy, sometimes referred to as chi or prana.

For a single food to qualify as a "superfood," it must not only provide a wide spectrum of nutrients but also tangibly improve some aspect of your mental and/or physical capacity. That's why foods like oatmeal, grapes and acai berries, while good for you, do not rise to the level of superfoods.

The Superfood by Which All Others Are Measured

The food that best fits this description is called E3Live®, a fresh green superfood used by Olympic gold medalists and professional athletes for endurance and mental clarity. It is considered to be at the top of the pyramid of all superfoods by those who eat raw, fresh, pure, organic green foods. E3Live® has now become popular with Hollywood celebrities and is happily coming to the attention of the wider public. It is the *real* "Real Thing."

Dr. Brian Clement, director of the Hippocrates Health Institute in West Palm Beach, Florida, where wheatgrass was popularized, calls E3Live® "the most nutritious food on the planet." It is safe for everyone, including infants, elders, and pregnant women. E3Live® offers all the health benefits of wheatgrass, and many additional benefits, as well.

E3Live®, known by the aquabotanical name of *Aphanizomenon flos-aquae*, or AFA, is among the rarest food found on Earth! It is certified organic, wild-grown, and harvested only at Klamath Lake, in the Oregon high desert. It restores the body and turns it in the direction of health. This therapeutic superfood is truly a healing gift from God or, if you like, from Mother Nature. It is good to know that some things in this world are pure, good, and wholesome.

In personally evaluating numerous superfoods in my own practice over the years, I have come to recognize that E3Live® is the superfood by which all others are measured.

Why E3Live® Is At The Top of My List

Supplementing your diet with E3Live® is the fastest way I know to kick-start your return to health. I personally use it every day. It is teeming with enzymatic life and highly cleansing! It contains over 64 perfectly balanced, naturally occurring vitamins, minerals, amino acids (protein) and essential fatty acids and has nearly four times the chlorophyll of wheatgrass. E3Live® also has an extremely high assimilation rate of up to 90%.

E3Live® contains long-chain omega-3 fatty acids and an array of trace minerals, including germanium, gold, selenium, and zinc. It also sports 22 of the 24 amino acids, including all eight of the essential ones, in a proportion perfect for optimum utilization by humans. In fact, E3Live's amino acid profile is very similar to that of mother's milk.

Key Benefits

I avidly recommend this remarkable superfood to all my patients, particularly those recovering from or working with an active illness. In addition to its nutrient density, E3Live® is best known for the following health benefits:

- **Energy:** It provides an enduring and smooth energetic lift.
- **Clarity:** It enhances focus, attention, and mental clarity.
- **Joy:** It is anti-depressive, balancing and uplifting mood. Its amino acid profile, and particularly the phenylalanine, supplies the neurotransmitter precursors that balance brain chemistry.
- **Purification:** Its high chlorophyll content purifies the body.
- **Immunity:** It stimulates white blood cells to ingest foreign particles and microorganisms.
- **Healing and repair:** It is the first natural compound known to stimulate stem cell release and migration, thus activating the body's innate healing, regeneration, and repair functions.
- **Blood sugar:** It helps stabilize blood sugar levels and as a result naturally decreases people's cravings for high-glycemic foods (refined sugars and starches). This decreases the inflammatory effects of these foods and also helps people reduce excess body fat.
- **Recovery time:** High-level athletes are able to increase training loads by reducing their recovery time.
- **Reduced inflammation:** Phycocyanin, the blue pigment in E3Live®, is a natural COX-2 selective inhibitor with strong anti-inflammatory properties.

In my own practice, I have seen E3Live® reverse premature aging as it eliminates toxins and repairs cell damage. My patients look and feel younger, and their moods are more stable, as well.

PEA — the "Love Molecule"

E3Live® contains naturally occurring phenylethylamine (PEA), a neurotransmitter that has demonstrated positive effects on sustaining mental attention and smoothing out mood. You may have heard the notion that chocolate makes you feel like you're in love. This is because chocolate contains PEA, commonly referred to as the "love molecule." When people are in love, their biochemistry shows higher amounts of PEA.

E3Live® happens to contain about fifty times more PEA than chocolate. This remarkable substance is exactly what promotes mental clarity and increased attention span, along with a sense of uplifted mood. University studies have shown that PEA is reduced in the brains of depressed patients.

Purification

Chlorophyll is a powerful purifier, and E3Live® has significantly more chlorophyll than wheatgrass, spirulina, or chlorella. Chemistry professor Karl Abrams says, "E3Live® contains more bioavailable chlorophyll than any other food. In biochemical research circles, the presence of chlorophyll in such high quantities is a clear indication of E3Live's extraordinarily high life force. This inherent vitality helps keep E3Live's wide spectrum of nutrients at their absolute nutritional peak. For me, this partially explains the mystery of how E3Live® can have so many positive health benefits."

Let's look at a few of the many benefits of chlorophyll:

1. It helps to detoxify the body, especially of heavy metals like mercury.

2. It delivers magnesium and helps the blood carry oxygen to cells and tissues.

3. Along with vitamins such as A, C, and E, it has been shown to help neutralize free radicals that damage healthy cells.

4. It is an effective deodorizer that reduces bad breath, as well as urine, fecal, and body odors.

5. It may reduce the ability of carcinogens to bind with the DNA in different major organs in the body.

Immunity

When it comes to healing and immune factors, taking a tablespoon of E3Live® daily has been shown to stimulate the migration of NK (natural killer) cells from the blood to the tissues. NK cells are known to be scavengers and killers of cancer and virally infected cells. E3Live® is the only known natural food to contain a unique polysaccharide that has been shown to stimulate the activity of macrophages (white blood cells that ingest foreign particles and infectious microorganisms).

A Superfood for Children Too!

If you want your children to eat well, add some E3Live® to their favourite juice. When children eat fast-food burgers or snacks, they become addicted to the combination of fried oil and salt, fried oil and sugar, or both — and they generally do not enjoy the taste of fresh vegetables. However, E3Live® is like the anti-Big Mac. When children (or adults) drink E3Live®, their sense of taste shifts, and healthy fruits and vegetables become appealing. They naturally want to eat better!

Smoothie Recipe and E3Live® Instructions

Here are some guidelines for incorporating E3Live® into your daily regimen:

Phase One

When introducing E3Live® into your diet, it is important to start slowly and follow these recommendations closely to ensure best results.

Adding E3Live® to a good-tasting smoothie makes all the difference! Please invest in a good quality blender if you don't already own one. Then buy a few bananas and either some fresh or frozen berries or some sweet ripe pineapple (make sure the latter two are organic, as both berries and pineapple are heavily sprayed with toxic chemicals when grown conventionally). Take the time to chop the bananas and pineapple into small chunks, and freeze them in sealed containers. This way, you will have fresh fruit readily available to blend each morning.

Blend the following until smooth, and then add E3Live®:

- 8 oz. apple or orange juice
- 2 tablespoons frozen pineapple
- One half frozen banana, or 2 tablespoons of frozen berries

If you have been eating a primarily vegetarian or vegan diet with a high percentage of fruits and vegetables, you can start with one tablespoon a day for the first five days and increase to two tablespoons a day for the next five days.

If you have been eating a lot of flesh, dairy, processed and refined junk food, and the like, then start by adding one teaspoon a day to your smoothie for five days. Then increase the dosage every five days, progressing from two teaspoons to one tablespoon, to two tablespoons a day. After that, add one tablespoon per week, until you reach four to five tablespoons.

Drink your smoothie first thing in the morning on an empty stomach, and wait at least 20 minutes before eating anything else (other than fruit). On an empty stomach, E3Live® in a fruit smoothie is rapidly absorbed into the bloodstream. It is best not to take the smoothie after a heavy or starchy meal.

It is important to stay hydrated and drink at least six to eight glasses of clean water a day, especially when introducing E3Live®.

Phase Two

After you have progressed to a week with four or five tablespoons of E3Live®, it's time to enter Phase Two, in which you take a second dose of E3Live® each morning. Ideally, I recommend that all my patients limit themselves to two solid meals a day (an early lunch and dinner), eating only fruit or liquids (E3Live® smoothies, herb teas, freshly squeezed juices) prior to lunch.

If you are very athletic and train at least an hour a day, or if you are vegetarian, you can drink a second smoothie with two tablespoons of E3Live® immediately following training in the morning, or you can take it to work in a thermos and drink it midmorning.

All others may take one teaspoon in a second smoothie mid-afternoon for five days then increase to one tablespoon for another five days. You may then proceed to two tablespoons in your second smoothie.

I recommend that most people continue at this level for four to eight weeks and work on making other healthy improvements in their lives. Examples include getting more exercise, exploring restorative stretching, drinking more water, eating more fresh organic produce, and decreasing the amount of refined junk foods they consume.

Phase Three

After a month or two, start experimenting with setting aside one day a week where you either fast on E3Live® and fresh juice until the next morning or alternatively until dinner, at which time you limit your first meal to fresh fruit, a salad, or a fresh, homemade vegetable soup. After that, you can return to your normal dietary program.

Professional athletes who train for a minimum of two hours a day can now start taking larger doses. I suggest experimenting with four to five tablespoons in a smoothie before and after training. Others can increase the second smoothie to three tablespoons.

Phase Four

When daylong fasts have become a routine part of your week, you can progress to Phase Four, in which you are encouraged to experiment with longer fasts, lasting from one to three days, from time to time.

On those days, eat only fruit (fresh, juiced, or blended), vegetable juice, or blended vegetable soups, with up to three doses per day of E3Live® (3 to 4 tablespoons at a time). Fasting with E3Live® and fresh juices is a great way to accelerate your detoxification and rejuvenation process.

For More Information

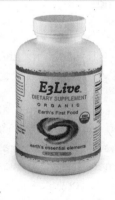

E3Live® Aquabotanical: You can buy this product on my website. Visit www.RenewYourself.net and click E3Live® in the navigation panel at left or view under Supplements.

E3Live® BrainON®

E3Live® BrainON® is a sister product to E3Live®, to which an additional water-soluble extract of E3Live® has been added. This additional extract contains extra amounts of PEA. E3Live® BrainON® is particularly suitable for those seeking to maximize attention and mental focus and to balance their moods.

The Only Healthy, Effective Natural Antidepressant

Dr. Gabriel Cousens, an integrative medicine MD with a degree in psychiatry, recommends nontoxic E3Live® and E3Live® BrainON® to patients suffering from depression, over and above popular prescription antidepressants with their unhealthy side effects. Dr. Cousens states, "E3Live® and E3Live® BrainON® offer specific benefits to the nervous system and brain function. It also has an expansive effect on our consciousness. More than any other food, E3Live® enables us to make a paradigm shift and enjoy a sense of well-being. Many people experience a quality of joy that's really subtle with E3Live® BrainON®."

Remarkably, he relates, "I've had people who've been depressed for years and years, and literally, within a few days after receiving E3Live® BrainON®, their depression lifts. This is because E3Live® gets to the root of helping heal the addictive brain chemistry that underlies a lot of depression."

Dr. Cousens emphasizes that we do not have a Prozac deficiency! We likewise suffer no lack of Lexapro, Effexor, Cymbalta, or Paxil. Millions of ordinary people could discard their toxic antidepressant drugs and achieve comparable (often superior) results with E3Live® BrainON® — while boosting their overall health at the same time!

All pharmaceutical drugs do us harm, damaging the heart, liver, kidneys, and other organs, and compromising our well-being and vitality in countless ways. Eliminating the need for pharmaceuticals is always the healthiest option.

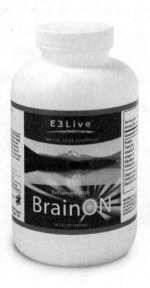

Pure Synergy

This is a true story. Mitchell May was involved in a serious car accident a ways back. His leg was broken in 42 pieces and sustained extensive vascular damage. Seventy different UCLA surgeons looked at Mitchell's leg and thought it should be amputated. Mitchell opted for a way to heal, and pursued non traditional methods. It was during this time that Mitchell developed Pure Synergy. He lived on Pure Synergy for a long time and did energy medicine. He now runs regularly.

In my opinion it is the number one powdered green food out there.

It contains 4 kinds of algaes, and several kinds of seaweed. It has a has over 8 kind of sprouts with lots of enzymes, and Chinese super herbs extracts, including reishi, cordyceps, astragalus, and fo-ti. Reishi, cordyceps, and astragalus are considered among the most important supertonic herbs for protection, by their immune modulating effects. This means if your immune system is overactive with responses like allergies, lupus, and rheumatoid arthritis, the immune modulating effect would lower it. If your immune system is under active it will bring it up. Reishi mushroom has a calming and strengthening effect. Fo-ti replenishes our deep reserves of essence energy, known as our jing. Pure Synergy has freeze dried juice concentrates of wheatgrass, barley grass, oat grass, alfalfa grass, parsley, spinach, kale, and collards. It also has a number of western herbs many of which are blood purifiers and anti-oxidants; such as red clover, burdock root, yellow dock root, dandelion leaf, and ginko. In total is has over 64 superfoods, algaes, sprouts, grasses, and herbs in it.

There are scores of green powder drinks out there and I have tried many of them. Pure Synergy makes me feel great! When you look at the Kirlian photography of the products in Pure Synergy there are massive bright bioelectrical energy fields coming off each and every ingredient. All of the products are of the finest organic origin; there are no fillers. They are prepared and blended into the powder in a way that leaves them enzymatically and bioelectrically in tact with their life force. In the powdered form they are easily assimilated with juice on an empty stomach, and in the bloodstream within 20 minutes.

The Pure Synergy is so alive; you can feel the Life Force. The powder tastes good and gives one a great feeling of energy and mental clarity. I recommend it as the number two supplement people add to their diet after E3Live®. When combined with fresh vegetable juicing you are flooding your body with light and Super Nutrients that are easily digested. Pure Synergy is also available in veggie capsules. Pure Synergy veggie caps are excellent to have in the car or at work for emergencies.

If you are under a lot of stress, or really depleted you may want to take some Men's or Women's Vita Synergy whole food multivitamins. They are loaded with vitamins, minerals, and lots of herbs.

For More Information

Pure Synergy: Visit www.RenewYourself.net and click on the supplements tab.

Natural Cellular Defense

In exams performed by the Red Cross on babies, a total of 287 chemicals were found in the baby's blood; 180 are known to cause cancer, 217 are toxic to the brain and nervous system, and 208 cause birth defects in animals.

As Gabriel Cousens M.D. has revealed in interviews, immune systems are compromised by lifestyles and toxic exposure. Some estimates show that as much as 25% of Americans suffer from some level of heavy metal poisoning; mercury, lead, cadmium, and arsenic are the most common. Chernobyl and the depleted uranium bombs of the Iraq War are two examples of our increasing exposure to harmful radiation.

Natural Cellular Defense:

- Uses zeolites to encapsulate and eliminate heavy metals- mercury, lead, cadmium, arsenic, herbicides, furans, and dioxins
- Activates the P21 tumour suppressing gene
- Blocks virus production
- Inactivates and eliminates free radicals
- Has a mildly alkalizing effect on over acid systems
- Has an immune system modulating effect
- Helps to reduce radioactive contamination

Because the zeolites in the natural cellular defense encapsulate the toxins that they are eliminating, the process is very smooth. Dr. Cousens has used the product successfully with pregnant women. When you do other methods of chelation for heavy metals, it is not always smooth, and can be costly. When doing EDTA chelation, I experienced very heavy mercury detox symptoms. I started breaking out in sweats, and feeling feverish during sleep. In contrast the NCD has always been very smooth.

On the subject of heavy metal poisoning, it's only fair to discuss the subject of amalgam fillings. If you have amalgam fillings you need to get them taken out by a qualified dentist and replaced with porcelain as soon as possible!

If you have any questions on why I am saying this, please watch the 5-minute video in the "For More Information" section. **THIS IS A MUST SEE!** Once you have the fillings out you need to take Natural Cellular Defense!

You should be aware of the radioactive contamination that we are all being exposed to. The smart bombs that the U.S. used in Iraq were made of depleted uranium. When the bombs vaporized upon detonation the radioactive particles went up into the lower atmosphere. We all now have to deal with the effects of this. It is concentrated most heavily in the upper end of the food chain. Meat and dairy concentrate radioactivity along with other environmental toxins. Water is another source of contamination. When we are being exposed to a lot of environmental toxicity it is even more important that we eat at the bottom of the food chain to minimize exposure.

For More Information

Natural Cellular Defense: Visit www.RenewYourself.net and click on the supplements tab. Take NCD to protect against radioactive contamination.

Smoking Teeth = Poison Gas: http://iaomt.org/videos/ Five-minute video about mercury silver fillings by the International Academy of Oral Medicine and Toxicology.

Probiotics

A proper balance of intestinal flora is absolutely essential for health. When you undergo antibiotic therapy you not only kill off pathological microbes, but all the positive flora in your intestine as well. It is imperative that you start probiotic supplementation to reinnoculate your colon. I feel it is a good idea to take probiotics daily, at regular intervals. Here is a list of some of their benefits:

- They contribute to the destruction of moulds, viruses, fungus, and parasites.
- They help maintain healthy cholesterol and triglyceride levels.
- They improve immune function.
- They protect against environmental toxins.
- They reduce toxic waste at a cellular level.
- They break down plaque build-up in the colon.
- They help manufacture vitamins B_1, B_2, B_3, B_6, B_{12}, and vitamins A and K.
- They cleanse the intestinal tract, purify the colon, and promote regular bowel movements.
- They contribute to a useful weight-loss program.

The best way to integrate a healthy intestinal flora culture to your GI tract is by consuming raw cultured vegetables such as sauerkraut. They are available in the refrigerated section of your health-food store. The other option is by making coconut water kefir. By buying young coconut water and adding a good kefir culture to it while at room temperature you can have a good culture in 24 hours. Drink a half to one cup a day. It can take up to months of regularly consuming these products with a healthy diet to fully cultivate a healthy culture in your GI tract.

For More Information

Click on Supplements section at www.RenewYourself.net.

Triphala

Triphala is one of the oldest tonics and rejuvenates. It is gentle and balancing for all body types. Triphala is specific for eliminating Ama and cholesterol from the body. Ama is a term denoting a substance associated with chronic disease patterns and symptoms of ageing. It is described as a kind of sticky build-up of material that clogs the circulatory channels.

In many ways it is nearly identical to the accumulation of excess cholesterol and blood lipids described in the West. Both conditions seem to contribute to a wide variety of circulatory disorders ranging from senility, rheumatic conditions, and cancer to heart disease.

Triphala is a completely balanced energetic formula, being neither too cold, nor too hot. When taken regularly over a long period, it gently effects the elimination and purification of Ama from the tissues of the entire body. The three fruits that comprise it (harada, amla, and bihara) have been scientifically studied and confirm some of its known traditional benefits. These include the lowering of cholesterol, reducing high blood pressure, benefiting circulation, improving digestion and regulating elimination without causing any laxative dependency. As a result, it is regarded as a kind of universal panacea.

A popular folk saying in India is, "No mother? Do not worry so long as you have Triphala." The reason being, that Triphala is able to care for the internal organs of the body as a mother cares for her children.

Generally the dose is from two to six capsules taken one to three times daily. A smaller dose might be one or two capsules three times a day. One should increase or decrease the dose according to one's bowel movements. Since there are no problems in using Triphala, the dose can be adjusted upwards or downwards from the suggested amount.

For More Information

Triphala: Visit www.RenewYourself.net and click the supplements tab.

Chinese Super Tonic Herbs

Chinese super tonic herbs form another category. Many of the medicinal mushrooms and other super tonic herbs contain extremely potent immune system modulators, strengthen the Life essence, build vitality (qi), and balance the spirit. These herbs are effective when obtained from a reputable source, where the potency, purity, and preparation are intact and taken properly over a long period of time.

In Chinese herbalism, there exists a special class of herbs that goes beyond the standard ones that treat symptoms or rebalance organs. These herbs are known as the Chinese super tonic herbs.

If taken over a long period of time, they help produce a state of health that supports increased longevity. They are important and unique enough that they form a separate food group by themselves. The super tonic herbs are very nutritious and can be taken under any circumstances. They strengthen and balance the organs and systems of the body. The body becomes more adaptable and experiences less wear and tear.

Chinese Herbalism uses the Three Treasure System of Healthcare. Ron Teegaurden uses the following analogy of life being like a candle to understand the Three Treasures Concept.

- The candle itself — the wax and wick — form the essence of the candle. Depending on the quality of wax and size of the candle, it can be expected to have a certain life. The candle is analogous to our jing.

- The flame is the activity of the candle. It provides the source of light, but eventually consumes the candle. The flame is like our qi.

- The light given off by the flame is the ultimate purpose of the candle. A larger candle thus a larger flame will give off greater light. The light given off by the candle is like shen, which is our spirit.

Our lives are like that of a candle. Genetically we are given certain regenerative power, but when our jing is used up we die. The purpose of taking Chinese super tonic herbs is to replenish the jing and qi and to stabilize our emotional body so that shen may fully develop.

- The first treasure, jing, is your deep seated essence or Life Force. When you are trying to build jing you must try to stop the Leaks. Jing is leaked by excessive stress, drug use, exhaustion, overwork, chronic illness, child birth, and worrying. Most westerners are jing deficient.

- The second treasure is known as qi. It is our vitality and is acquired thru breathing and eating. It affects our digestive, respiratory and immune functions, and helps us to adapt to stress. Many Qi tonics include Reishi mushrooms because of their strong immune modulating effects, and adaptogens like Ginseng and Gynostemma.

- The third treasure is our shen, or spirit. It is said to be the divinity that resides in our hearts. Negative emotions stunt shen. Giving and service help to build shen, along with taking shen-building herbs. Taking reishi mushrooms over a long period of time will build shen.

The average person is so depleted he/she needs to do a program with the following Super Tonic Herbal combinations for 100 days just to begin to build a foundation of health.

Treasure Pack Tonic Herbal Program

The following four products are sold as a package, and can be taken by men and women, of all ages:

- **He Shou Wu Formulation:** This is a jing tonic and enriches kidney yin. This formula is headed by Polygonum. It is a superb anti-ageing and rejuvenation formula.

- **Super Adaptive:** If you could take just one formula, this would be it. It is a full spectrum adaptogen formula that nourishes all three treasures. Adaptogens help us deal with stress and stimulate the body's own immune and healing functions. Super Adaptogen contains many of the most potent herbs in the world.

- **Supreme Protector:** This formulation is composed of the three kings of defense in Chinese herbalism: reishi, astragalus, and cordyceps. All protect the body, mind, and spirit in various ways. Each is a potent immune modulator and all have powerful antioxidant and anti-stress properties. The herbs help protect the liver from toxins and the lungs from pollutants, while strengthening the kidneys and adrenals. In addition, it powerfully tonifies all three treasures.

- **Spring Dragon Gynostemma Longevity Tea:** Made from Gynostemma pentaphillum, one of the top ten herbs in the world, Spring Dragon Gynostemma is an all-natural green tea that contains no caffeine. It has 82 phytochemicals similar to those in ginseng. It enhances immune function, serves as an adaptogen, and soothes inflammation. It's a good tasting tea and one should drink of it freely on a daily basis.

I would like to give credit to Ron Teegaurden of Dragon Herbs for a majority of the information in the Chinese Super Tonic Herb section. Ron's website www.dragonherbs.com is a beautiful website with a wealth of information. If you are interested in learning more about Chinese super tonic herbs, this is a great place to start. Dragon Herbs also offers a beautiful free catalogue that provides additional information.

For More Information

Treasure Pack Program: Visit Error! Hyperlink reference not valid. on the Supplements tab.

Additional Supplements

A number of other natural supplements are available that possess tremendous healing properties. I will briefly highlight additional supplements that I have found to be the most beneficial.

Enzymes

Enzymes are the "spark" of life. Without enzymes, our bodies do not properly break down food; therefore we don't absorb vitamins, minerals, and amino acids which are the basis of health. Our immune system, bloodstream, liver, kidneys, spleen and especially pancreas depend upon enzymes for proper digestive function. Without proper enzymes, our white blood cells try to perform the purpose of the enzymes, usually leaving one feeling tired after eating, and compromising the immune system. Enzymes are responsible for every biochemical reaction that occurs in living matter. All life depends on enzymes.

Digestive enzymes tend to decrease as we get older. Eating cooked and over processed foods compounds this situation... Enzymes in food are rendered inactive by cooking above 118 degrees.

Enzymes can be used to decrease the inflammatory response and speed recovery from injuries. Bromelain is used a lot with professional athletes to speed recovery from sports injuries. Enzymes can also be used with patients in acute or chronic pain. When using enzymes for these reasons they are best taken between meals, one to two capsules every hour. People with ulcers should check with their doctors.

Aloe Vera

Aloe-Vera has high concentrations of polysaccharides that modulate the immune system and contains large amounts of prana or life force. It is cleansing and anti-inflammatory. The juice has a high amount of ormus containing mono atomic minerals and lots of energy.

Ormus is a topic for a whole discussion in itself. One of the leading researchers in this area is David Wolfe. Click www.thebestdayever.com to listen to archives of audio and video lectures.

It is now possible to buy live organic aloe vera juice. I recommend adding a tablespoon of this to your super smoothie. The best idea would be to have aloe vera plants growing in your garden and home, and to filet the leaves, and add the gel to your smoothies.

The aloe vera is also excellent to apply to the skin. It has a tonifying effect on loose skin. It is excellent on the face and great for itching and burns on the skin.

Maca

Maca is like Peruvian ginseng. It is an adaptogen and has a balancing effect on the endocrine system, particularly the thyroid. It increases, stamina, energy, heat, and the ability to deal with stress. It may need to be curtailed during hot summer months.

Bee Pollen and Royal Jelly

Bee pollen and royal jelly both contain extraordinary amounts of prana or life force. They are very nutrient dense. Both should be from organically certified sources and raw and refrigerated in dark sealed bottles.

Both bee pollen and royal jelly are considered extreme longevity foods and tonics. There are references to the high percentage of Georgian Centurions that were bee keepers and daily partook of honey, pollen and royal jelly.

Bee Pollen contains high amounts of choline. Choline drops by 40% in long distance runners. Competitive swimmers are able to swim longer without exhaustion when adding choline to their nutrient intake. Learn more about this natural miracle food and start adding it to your super smoothie.

I would rank bee pollen and royal jelly as being the third and fourth most important supplement to add to your daily regime.

Raw Hempseeds

Organic hulled hempseeds are rich in Omega 3 fatty acids, and have an easy to digest form of protein called edastin. It makes a good addition to super smoothies. Hemp is over 30% easy to digest protein. It is also high in fibre.

Hemp is high in choline, inositol, and lecithin, which are great for the nervous system. Hemp has a 1:3 ratio of omega 3's to Omega 6's. Hemp seeds supply about 2% GLA (gamma linoleic acid), which is important in the eicosanoid pathways. The hemp plant root system goes about 10 feet deep picking up many trace minerals.

Goji Berries

Goji berries should be a staple in your diet. They have been associated with longevity in many Chinese healing traditions. Chinese medicine considers them to be one of the 52 super tonic herbs.

Goji berries offer the following benefits:

- They have a high concentration of rejuvenating polysaccharides.
- They are low on the glycemic index.
- They are high in antioxidants, as evidenced by their deep red color.
- They contain a good balance of all eight essential amino acids.
- They create an environment conducive to optimum HGH (human growth hormone) release.

Be sure the berries are organic. I recommend snacking on them and using them in fruit salads. You should be eating one half to one cup a day.

Himalayan Crystal Salt

The right kind of salt is absolutely essential. Ordinary table salt is 97.5 per cent sodium chloride plus some chemicals heated to 1200 degrees. It is a poison. Every gram the body cannot get rid of requires 23 grams of water to neutralize. It stresses the kidneys and aggravates arthritic type conditions.

Pink Himalayan salt crystals contain 84 trace minerals in a crystalline form, which allows the body to re-establish homeostasis. It acts as a catalyst in the uptake of other nutrients. It is not toxic like table salt. All table salt should be discarded and replaced with Himalayan Crystal Salt immediately.

Athletes and people training hard should add small amounts of this salt to their diet, particularly those in hot climates for avoiding dehydration.

These salts contain calcium, magnesium, potassium, and sodium which maintain electrolyte balance. These minerals are crucial for athletes to prevent dehydration, electrolyte imbalance and cramping.

A pinch of Himalayan salt with young coconut water, E3Live®, fresh squeezed celery juice, a dab of coconut oil and a teaspoon of raw monuka honey would be an excellent blend to stay hydrated on for multiple competitive heats in a hot sunny climate. Drinking fresh squeezed green vegetable juices during training will also help with dehydration.

Pink Himalayan salt crystals are also ideal for brine baths. When done in the right concentration they have a very therapeutic effect. The right concentration would be about 2.5 lbs of bath crystals for an average 30 gallon bath tub. Soak for 20-30 minutes and dry off without showering. The Bath should be plenty warm. If you have any type of heart condition, cancer, diabetes, or circulatory problems you need to check with your medical doctor as always before initiating this procedure. The bath will pull toxins out of the body thru osmosis. The detoxifying effect of a Salt Bath can be compared to a 3 Day Fast. It will loosen up stiff and over contracted muscles. Have some pink salt lamps in the bathroom, to generate negative ions.

After soaking in the bath is an excellent time to have a green drink or hot herbal tea, followed by some restorative stretches, and breathing exercises.

Omega Essential Fatty Acids

About 90 percent of the general population have a deficiency in Omega 3 fatty acids, especially the long chain omega 3 fatty acids, EPA (eicosapentaenoic acid) and DHA (docohexaenoic acid). The balance of Omega 6s to Omega 3s should be about 3 to 1. Omega 3s and particularly the long branched EPA and DHA exert a powerful anti-inflammatory and mood elevating effect. They are an important part of the brain and nervous system.

Omega-3s are available in organic raw flax seed powder or oil and hemp seed. EPA and DHA are available in E3Live® Aquabotanical, as well as micro distilled fish and krill oil.

I recommend initially that people add a teaspoon of flax powder to their smoothies. The flax will also supply much needed additional fibre and act as an intestinal broom. I additionally recommend one teaspoon of hemp seed oil, and one teaspoon of raw coconut oil. You will read more about these later.

For those people that are feeling depressed and are in chronic pain, I recommend initially supplementing with a micro-distilled brand of fish oil or krill oil that is rich in EPA and DHA. The therapeutic dose can be up to four 1000mg. capsules a day. I don't recommend buying fish oils from the health food store unless microdistilled. Microdistilled krill oil is also very excellent.

Having the right balance of EFAs speeds up fat metabolism. They are precursors of many hormones, and help with recovery from workouts, modulate blood sugar levels, are anti-inflammatory, and mood elevating.

It is important to reduce or eliminate cooked fats. Most processed foods contain highly carcinogenic trans fatty acids (shown on food labels with the words "hydrogenated" or "partially hydrogenated"). This includes all crisps, fried food, biscuits, cakes, cookies, crackers, pretzels, donuts, commercial peanut butter, margarine, and meat.

These need to be replaced with good oils like hemp seed, coconut oil, avocados, olives, and the EPA and DHA that are in E3Live®. The percentage of oil that you personally need will depend on your body type, the time of year, and where you live.

Coconut Oil

Coconut oil is up to 50% medium chain saturated fatty acids which have anti-viral, anti-fungal, and anti-microbial properties. Raw organic coconut oil has a stimulating effect upon thyroid function and lowers cholesterol levels. In the presence of proper thyroid function LDL cholesterol is converted to the anti-ageing hormones pregnenolone, progesterone, and DHEA.

When cattle ranchers added coconut oil to the cattle diet in hopes of increasing their weight they were very shocked! The cows actually lost weight. Studies have indicated that adding Coconut Oil to the diet over a six week period of time may raise the bar on endurance type athletic endeavours. Small amounts of raw coconut oil in the diet helps to stabilize blood sugar levels, and insulin receptor sensitivity.

Young Coconut Water

The water from young Thai coconuts is low in fat and high in minerals. It is very hydrating, cooling, and tastes slightly sweet. It is called the Fluid of Life due to the similarity of its mineral content and composition to blood plasma.

When you combine it with a top quality live green superfood like E3Live® or pure synergy, you have a blood transforming drink. The haemoglobin molecule in the blood is almost identical to the chlorophyll molecule. The difference is, the chlorophyll molecule has magnesium in the center and the haemoglobin molecule has iron in the center.

Young coconut water is an excellent base for smoothies, green drinks, and fasting. In climates or locations where it may be difficult to procure top quality produce for making fresh juices, coconut water is a great alternative. It is an excellent drink for athletes to be drinking during training and competition, because it helps to re-hydrate and replenish electrolytes.

Manuka Honey

Raw organic Manuka honey is a natural antibiotic, one of the highest prana foods, and has powerful immune boosting properties supported by a substantial body of scientific research. It is high in anti-oxidents, contains health promoting pro-biotics, and is a more natural and endurance enhancing solution for your sweet tooth. It is harvested from a pristine area of New Zealand where the bees gather their pollen almost exclusively from the Manuka bush.

Cacao

Cacao is where chocolate comes from, it is the raw chocolate bean. It has very powerful anti-oxidant properties. It enhances the production of Anandamide, one of the bliss chemicals in the brain, as well as PEA (phenylethylamine), the molecule of love. Cacao is high in magnesium, which by the way is deficient in a majority of the population. Cacao is enhanced when combined with E3Live® and BrainON®.

Commercial chocolate is heated and processed with bad fats and sugars. Cacao is actually good for you. Some great cacao chocolate bars with all natural ingredients are now being made. Cacao has re-emerged recently in the west, due largely to the efforts of David Wolfe. David and Shazzie have written an excellent book on Cacao called *Naked Chocolate.*

For More Information

Visit Error! Hyperlink reference not valid. on the Vivapura tab.

PART 4: HEALTHY PRODUCTS

Keetsa Mattresses

Sleep is the foundation of good health. And quality sleep provides the body an opportunity to rebuild and prepare for the assault of a new day. If your bed is not comfortable and supportive, if your sleep environment is not conducive to sleep, you could spend 8 hours of restless sleep and not get what your body needs. An integral part of proper sleep is a healthy, supportive mattress.

Keetsa is a company that produces a mattress which addresses the proper support our bodies need though using affordable non-toxic, recycled, and organic materials. Most major brand mattresses rely heavily on synthetic materials such as polyester fabrics, poly-fills and petroleum based foams that can represent an off-gassing nightmare. These mattress companies are not always very forthcoming about their ingredients. Keetsa takes pride in giving you all the information you need to make a smart choice.

Keetsa memory foam is made from 20% plant oil, reducing the dependency on synthetic materials. Keetsa uses a non-toxic fire barrier that complies with the Federal Fire Standards. Their memory foam also goes through a process that greatly reduces the off-gassing typical of most brands.

The Keetsa line of mattresses are very durable, and come with a 20 year warranty. Keetsa memory foam mattresses can be shipped directly to your home compressed in a biodegradable bag, vacuum sealed, and rolled in a box that you can put in your car.

Keetsa mattresses give you value and peace of mind, and most importantly, a great night's sleep!

For More Information

For more on Keetsa mattresses visit www.RenewYourself.net.

Om Gym

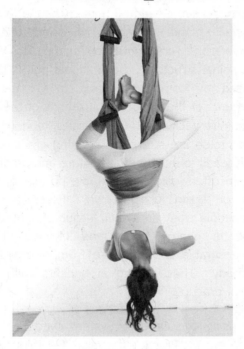

The OmGym Suspension System is a masterful tool to help maximize rejuvenation and longevity. Its adjustable design dramatically works to improve the anatomical structure and physiological health of all body types. It is a portable, cushioned yoga sling with a series of handles designed to assist, support, modify, and challenge the body where appropriate, through a huge variety of postures and exercises. Gravity is used as a tool to create patterns of healthy functionality. Users of the OmGym System can easily develop strength and flexibility without the need for a gym. With even a basic routine, it will greatly assist with detoxification, postural correction, and mood regulation. The OmGym System was presented on "The View" as "the number one natural remedy for depression."

A daily inversion therapy practice with your OmGym System is a great place to start. Inversion is an ancient secret of youth for mind and body. It increases blood supply and nutrient exchange to the brain, thyroid, pituitary, and pineal gland. Hanging inversion offers traction that decompresses the vertebrae, creating space for the discs while straightening and balancing the spinal structure. Gravitational pull is the easiest way to ease strains caused by compression and to lift the weight off the superimposed segments of the torso. Subluxations of the vertebrae tend to ease, helping to diminish back pain. The muscles, tendons, and ligaments of the entire back and torso are stretched, creating great feelings of opening and releasing. This leads to much better posture and greater spinal mobility. The OmGym System offers easy, comfortable positioning to help reap the amazing benefits of being upside-down. Results are often noticed immediately. Most people enjoy an overall feeling of lightness and elongation, along with a gentle energy boost and elevated mood after each session. These pleasurable feelings arise from biological changes taking place within the body. These biological benefits will become long-term effects with a regular practice.

I recommend using the OmGym System everyday with a variety of techniques that you enjoy. Practice inversion 1-4 minutes three times per day; once after waking, once before dinner, and immediately before bedtime. Choose 3-4 exercises to do along with inversion at each session for noticeable changes in all areas of body functionality.

Ultimate physical health begins with a healthy spinal column. As the posture corrects, so does the psychological well-being. When we are more balanced and neutral in position, the body can move with more efficiency and grace. Correcting posture also adds to confidence and feelings of self love. The OmGym is your lifeline to great postural variation. Begin in your comfort zone. The secret to longevity is creating life-long, pleasurable, and healthy habits. It is the love of journey that is important, not the destination!

For More Information

Visit www.RenewYourself.net and click on Neck and Back Health.

Essentia Mattresses and Pillows

Essentia makes the world's only natural memory foam mattresses and pillows. Why is this a big deal? Memory foam mattresses are known for their comfort, but they are far from healthy. These mattresses can contain up to 61 chemicals, including the carcinogens benzene and naphthalene.

When a family member was diagnosed with cancer, Jack Dell'Accio, the founder of Essentia, became aware of the many carcinogenic toxins found in everyday products. Jack's family had been in the latex foam business for years and supplied most major mattress brands. He realized that these mattresses were manufactured with poor quality components, filled with toxic foams, treated with harsh chemicals and layered together with glue.

Essentia mattresses are now the natural, non-toxic, and healthy alternative to Tempurpedic without compromising comfort. Essentia spent eight months creating their own organic cover when they learned that the industry's top certified organic cover contained polyester. Essentia even created a molding process which eliminates the need for glues. Now even the coloring used to create their signature stripe is organic. All Essentia mattresses are covered with their Zebrano fabric, an unbleached organic cotton cover with organic fill, organic backing and organic dyes.

It's clear for Essentia, mattresses are much more than something we sleep on. They're about proper blood circulation, spinal alignment, disk re-hydration all the while using natural materials for the healthiest possible sleep environment.

All Essentia mattresses are handmade made in Canada, come with a 20 year warranty, 60 day money back guarantee and they offer free shipping across North America.

For More Information

Visit www.RenewYourself.net to find out more about Essentia mattresses.

Earthing Conductive Bed Sheets

I have always felt a greater connection to the Earth and a certain invigorating energy walking barefoot. In fact walking barefoot goes far beyond a level of mere invigoration to actual physical healing.

Science has discovered that the surface of the Earth is brimming with an unlimited supply of free electrons that creates a gentle and undulating signal, stronger during the day and quieter at night. This electrical signal parallels the circadian rhythm of day and night and, as it turns out, may be a missing link to health, healing, and even longevity.

When connected to the Earth, either by being barefoot outside or sleeping at night on specially designed bed sheets connected to a ground rod outside or plugged into a properly grounded wall outlet, the free electrons flow into the body. We become instantaneously reconnected to a primordial signal that generates multiple benefits. Here is a short list of them:

- Defuses inflammation, and improves or eliminates the symptoms of many inflammation-related disorders.
- Reduces or eliminates chronic pain.
- Improves sleep in most cases.
- Increases energy.
- Lowers stress and promotes calmness in the body by cooling down the nervous system and stress hormones.
- Normalizes the body's biological rhythms.
- Thins blood, and improves blood pressure and flow.
- Relieves muscle tension and headaches.
- Lessens menopausal and menstrual symptoms.

The discovery of these, and other life-nurturing benefits, is documented in a fascinating book entitled *Earthing* (Basic Health Publications), written by Clinton Ober, cardiologist Stephen Sinatra, M.D., and Martin Zucker. For more than ten years, thousands of people around the world—men, women, children, and athletes—have incorporated Earthing into their daily routines. The results and their stories are extraordinary.

Throughout evolution, humans mostly walked the Earth barefooted, or in sandals made from hides (which are conductive), and slept on the ground. They didn't know it but they were receiving a daily dosage of natural healing energy from the Earth. This fascinating book explores the effect of the modern phenomenon of wearing footwear made from material that does not permit the conduction of the Earth's natural energy. In addition, sleeping in elevated beds means that few people regularly connect with the Earth's energy and therefore are missing the natural infusion of free electrons.

Separation from the Earth can cause chronic inflammation, now considered the main cause of many common and serious diseases, including cardiovascular and autoimmune diseases, cancer, and diabetes. Numerous anecdotes and growing scientific evidence demonstrates that physical reconnection with the Earth via going barefoot or sleeping on conductive bed sheets restores the healing signal and free electrons to the body.

I first heard about sleeping grounded in 2009 and obtained a conductive bed sheet. My experience has been positive. First I slept a lot more. Perhaps the Earth's energy was encouraging more rest, needed as a result of my very intense workload. Afterward, my sleep normalized but I've noticed that sleep is deeper than before. And my degree of energy remains as high as ever. I have heard many good things about sleeping grounded, including accounts from women whose PMS or menopausal symptoms have eased off or even disappeared. Based on the logic of this natural and evolutionary concept—connectedness with the Earth—I think you are going to hear a lot about *Earthing* in the future. I highly recommend the book.

This seems to me like another great—and surprising—lifestyle ingredient for restoring health and keeping yourself healthy for the long haul ahead.

For More Information

Earthing—conductive bed sheets: This product is available on my website. Visit www.RenewYourself.net.

Health Bridges

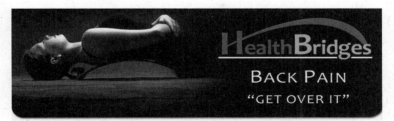

Photo courtesy of www.healthbridges.com

Many people complain of nagging aching pains in the middle and lower back. Without a regular stretching routing or hatha yoga practice, you can have a stiff and over-contracted middle back by your mid-thirties.

Slumping, poor posture, poor muscle tone and balance, can lead to chronically over contracted muscles in your middle back that cause long term postural deviations. After a decade or two of this, I often find that people have lost their ability to do extension in the mid-thoracic spine.

When I ask a person to arch his or her back, I often get an arching of the low back and neck, while the mid-back remains frozen in a forward bending flexed position. One of the most effective solutions for this is the Health Bridges Step system. The bridges come in three different templates or Steps, to allow us to gradually retrain the surrounding soft tissue.

Opening up the mid-back area can be a key to chronic back pain relief. This area has to be opened slowly and progressively on a daily basis. This is done by stretching your spine daily in forward bending, back bending, side-bending, and twisting. It took years for the damage to occur so be prepared for it to take time for your spine to regain its lost flexibility.

It may take several months of using Step One daily before you are ready to move onto Step Two. When you combine using these back boards or Bridges with deep breathing, detoxification, and restorative stretches, you have very powerful tools for affecting change quickly.

Traction Units

The spinal discs are avascular after the age of 12. Avascular tissue needs nutrition and waste product removal to function normally; as well as for repair and regeneration. Motion is what is needed to get nutrients moving in and waste products moving out. Therefore loading and unloading cycles should be started in both the cervical and lumbar spine as soon as possible. This is accomplished by cervical and lumbar intermittent traction.

The average person loses about 2 inches in height by the time he or she is 65, which can be attributed to degeneration and thinning of the inter-vertebral discs. These discs not only act as shock absorbers, they act as spacers for the holes that allow the spinal nerve trunks to exit the spinal column. These holes or foramina not only contain a nerve root, but a fat pad, artery, vein, and lymphatic. When the discs thin, the resulting thinning of the foramina can cause constriction of the nerve flow and circulation. If these compromised foramina are in the part of your neck that controls the nerves going down your arm, you may experience numbness, tingling, or pain in your arms and hands. If the foramina in question were controlling your sciatic nerve, you could experience sciatic pain in the buttocks or legs. By doing traction, not only do we help the discs, we relieve pressure and constriction on nerves and circulation. Additionally traction helps to relieve muscle spasms.

If you have chronic neck pain, headaches, tingling or pain in the arm, degenerative disc or degenerative joint disease, have been told by your doctor that you have "arthritis in your neck", and/or are over the age of 40, you probably will get huge benefit from doing home traction. For the neck we recommend the Pettibon home traction unit. It is inexpensive and can be done at home for 2-3 minutes several times a day.

For More Information

Visit www.RenewYourself.net and click on Neck and Back Health.

Orthotics

Today's orthotic should result from a weight bearing dynamic gait analysis. This is the information being gathered by a digitized gait and pressure analysis derived from walking over an electronic plate. The information is then sent to a lab over the internet. This is the system that pro-athletes in football and baseball and other sports use, and it represents a technological leap forward from the old style foam casting made and mailed to the lab.

If you have a rolling in of your foot (pronation) or a rolling out of your foot (supination) when you walk you may be a candidate for orthotics. You can also check to see if the heels of your shoes are wearing evenly. Correction of structural imbalances with your feet will save wear and tear on your knees, hips, and back over time.

For More Information

Footmaxx: www.footmaxx.com is an excellent place to get orthotics.

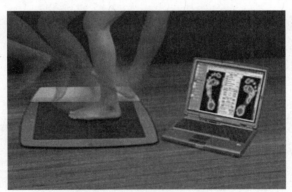

Photo courtesy of www.footmaxx.com

Human Touch Robotic Massage Chair

Who doesn't like a great massage? The reality of our high stressed life styles is that almost all of us could use a massage daily. The newest generation of the HT (Human Touch) Robotic massage chairs fits the bill perfectly. They are so good, that they actually feel better than some massage therapists. The HT-5040 not only gives a great massage from the neck to the soles of the feet, but is dependable and affordable. For $2300 you can have an attractive reclining massage chair delivered to your door step.

The Human Touch team of researchers analysed the treatment used by chiropractors and massage therapists and incorporated it into the most effective robotic massage chair on the market. They offer a variety of strokes that massage your neck and back, as well as your calves and feet. Besides hitting the large para-spinal muscle groups on both sides of your spine, they are also hitting all the acupuncture points associated with internal organs.

You can get a stunning back massage as often as you need. How good is it? Think Magical! Watch TV and get a daily massage that not only feels great, but is therapeutic. One of the best investments you could make in your health.

Add a far infrared pad, take Dr. Cromack's Super Smoothie, and put on the Holosync meditation program for a super rejuvenation session.

For More Information

Human Touch Robotic Chairs: Click the Human Touch Massage Chair tab at www.RenewYourself.net to see all five of the massage chairs.

SPECIAL COUPON! Enter the coupon code **HT400** at checkout to receive a $400 discount on any Human Touch Massage Chair.

Peter Ragnar and Magnetic Therapy

You may have noticed that Peter Ragnar is one of the four people I dedicated my book to. I consider Peter to be one of my mentors, and I hold him in very high esteem for many reasons.

Peter inspires me in many ways, and I feel that he has distilled down the essence of what works in terms of health and longevity. Peter doesn't talk about his age, because, as he says, "time is not toxic"; tearing off calendar pages has nothing to with personal performance and health. Besides a little white in his beard, Peter has aged remarkably little over the past thirty years.

In my opinion he is one of the strongest persons pound for pound of anybody on the planet any age. Some of his strength feats include bending steel horseshoes with his bare hands, performing 2000 dips in 80 minutes, pinch gripping 160 lbs. of weight plates with one hand, and leg pressing 2020 lbs. He has a 6th degree black belt in Shingitai Jujitsu. Peter is capable of extraordinary feats of mental focus and recall, is very successful, has a huge heart, and is very balanced.

Peter strongly advocates the use of magnetic therapy and, as a qi gong master, has successfully integrated the use of magnets with qi gong.

Magnetic Therapy

- 1989 Journal of the American Medical Association published an article entitled "Magnetism- A new method of stimulation for nerve and brain function". JAMA also referenced over 30 other articles in various medical journals.
- Dr. Gary Null's Book- **Healing with Magnets** references over 1000 peer reviewed articles on the benefits of magnetic therapy.
- The earth's magnetic field has decreased from a magnetic field of 4.0 at one time to .4 gauss presently.
- Electrical fields produce magnetic fields. The body has a bioelectrical

field that, when coupled with magnetic stimulation, enhances life span.

- The pineal gland has magnetite in it that responds to magnetic therapy.
- The most practical method of utilizing magnetic therapy is sleeping on a magnetic mattress pad.
- Sleeping on a magnetic mattress pad increases human growth hormone and melatonin production.
- Magnetic therapy has an alkalizing effect on the bloodstream, decreasing recovery time from heavy physical workouts.
- Decreases cell breakdown.
- Increases the body's ability to utilize oxygen.
- Has an overall anti-ageing and longevity effect.
- Avoid if pregnant or using a pacemaker.

I personally use his palm magnets and pineal gland magnets, along with the 3,950 gauss rare earth magnets for both my breathing and qi gong exercises. I did an interesting experiment the summer of 2009, and over several weeks graphed the chi flowing through my 12 acupuncture meridians upon rising and after magnetic breathing exercises, Magnetic Qi Gong, and again at the end of the day. Over a three week period of time, I had a several fold increase in the amount of chi moving through my acupuncture meridians as measured with electro meridian imaging. I also sleep with a magnetic mattress pad on my bed. Using a magnetic mattress pad is one of the easiest ways to integrate magnetic therapy into your health regime. I have had a substantial increase in my energy, well-being, and overall strength over the last 5 months of doing the breathing exercises and Magnetic Qi Gong exercises taught by Peter.

For More Information

Visit www.RenewYourself.net and click on the Peter Ragnar section.

Other Essential Tools for Health

In this section I have briefly listed a number of additional tools I see as essential for maintaining optimal health. I have always considered it a privilege to be able witness the health transformation for my patients when they realize the benefit of even some of these simple, but life-changing tools.

Far Infrared Saunas and Pads

Far infrared light penetrates six inches deep, allowing for detoxification of both the bloodstream and fat. A regular sauna or steam does not penetrate below the subcutaneous tissue. Far infrared clears blockages and restores flow to the entire microcirculatory system. It has the effect of

- Strengthening the immune system.
- Controlling pain.
- Improving cardiovascular function.
- Managing weight (burns 400 calories per half hour).
- Detoxifying heavy metals and other environmental toxins.

Saunas are a great way to utilize far infrared therapy at home. Far infrared mattress pads and chair pads are also available. They are made in a way that produces no electromagnetic interference, and they generate negative ions as well as amethyst crystal amplification of the far infrared. These pads are a perfect complement to top your Human Touch robotic massage chair.

Lumbar Supports

If you spend time sitting, you should be using a lumbar support in your car and at your desk. The problem is most of us slump after sitting for a while.

When you slump with your low back, your head moves anterior to your center of gravity. Your head weighs about ten to fourteen pounds. For every inch that your head translates forward of your center of gravity, the stress load upon your posterior neck muscles increases by about ten pounds. If this is going on a number of hours every day, there is a lot of stress being added, in the form of knots and spasms, in pain sensitive muscles.

These overcontracted and fatigued muscles can refer their own pattern in the form of myofascial pain syndromes. They are accompanied by trigger points, which are about the size of a quarter and tender.

If you want to be free of pain in your neck and back, then you must address ongoing postural stresses, and eliminate them.

Cervical Pillows

A healthy neck has a C-shaped curve from the side. This allows for optimal range of motion and distribution of the weight of the head, along the joints and discs in the neck. The normal pillow causes this curve to be reversed while you are sleeping and is orthopedically incorrect. The difference the correct pillow can make is significant. There are dozens of different cervical pillows out there and I have tried many of them. Some of them are uncomfortable. How do you find the right one?

The better pillows are made from memory-foam, and the Tempur-Pedic is among the best available. In the first few weeks of using the best orthopedic pillow, there may be some mild discomfort as your neck adapts to the correct support. After this initial adapting, I find it impossible to get a great night's sleep without my Tempur-Pedic cervical pillow. I take it with me when I travel. If you **are sensitive to foam** there are buckwheat pillows available that support a normal cervical curve.

For More Information

Visit www.renewyourself.net and click on Neck & Back Health.

Shower and Bath Filters

You should be using a shower filter to filter out the chlorine and other chemicals in your shower water. Your skin is the largest organ in the body, and readily absorbs whatever it is exposed to. This is how transdermal patches work.

The Waterwise Deluxe Showerwise effectively removes chlorine and other harmful contaminants. Your body can absorb more chlorine in a ten minute shower than from drinking the same water all day! It also reduces iron, lead, arsenic, mercury, hydrogen sulfide, several types of bacteria, algae, fungi and mold. Say goodbye to dull hair and irritated, itchy skin with Showerwise.

Water Purifiers

Simply, the water coming through our pipes isn't fit for consumption. I recommend putting a filter on your shower if you haven't already. There are numerous toxins in our water, which can include high levels of uranium.

The best solution at this time is to order a water distiller. The Waterwise Company has some inexpensive dependable distillers. The steam distillation process leaves only pure water. When you go to clean your distiller, you will be shocked at the amount of inorganic sediment. Seven gallons of distilling will leave one to two tablespoons of rock like sediment. This is not assimilated in your body, and in fact creates stiffness and clogging of the body.

Distilled water erases the energy signature of the water, so we are left with a clean slate. The water must then be restructured. This can be accomplished by any of the following:

- Adding crystal energy drops.
- Putting a crystal in a glass water jug and exposing it to moon light.
- Pouring the water thru something that creates a whirl pool vortex as the water passes over it.
- Adding gemstone elixirs.
- Adding a pinch of Himalayan Crystal Salt to a gallon of distilled water

and shaking.

By doing these things with distilled water you will notice that the water becomes "wetter". You need to be drinking 6-8 glasses of pure water per day, especially if you are taking NCD. The formula is about one ounce of water for every 2 pounds of body weight. You should be drinking your water warm, as it helps to flush away toxins from your digestive track. Ice cold water suspends digestion. Avoid it.

For More Information

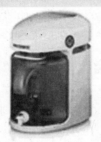

Photo courtesy of www.waterwise.com

Waterwise distillers: visit www.RenewYourself.net and click Appliances > Water Distillers in the navigation panel at left. The Model 9000 is pictured above. Click Contact to email me for a special discount coupon code on these products. I will get back to you promptly.

Air Purifiers

Unless you live on an island in the Pacific, or the Swiss Alps you should invest in an air purification system.

Most of us are spending a majority of our time indoors. Experts are voicing concerns that indoor pollution might be even more dangerous to our health than outdoor pollution.

"*Your home may be teaming with allergens such as dust, dander and pollens. Carbon monoxide can escape from fireplaces and gas stoves; upholstered furniture houses live dust mites, and pesticides emit toxic gases into the air. Mold and bacteria often funnel through heating, ventilation, and cooling systems and organic chemicals seep out of paints and carpets. Even common household products like air fresheners and cleaning agents can release pollutants continuously."* – The Airwise Company

"*Dust mites in the air cause allergic reaction in an estimated 15-20 percent of the population and have been linked to the development of childhood asthma.*"- Professor Yogi Goswami, Director of University of Florida Solar Energy, and Energy Conversion Laboratory

It's not a matter of whether you need an air treatment system, but which one you should chose. I like the Airwise Purifier; it goes way beyond HEPA, electrostatic, ozone, ultraviolet light, and negative ionizers. The Airwise technology uses photo catalysis to vaporize odors, fungi, mold, parasites, and toxic chemical gases. It significantly reduces allergens such as pollens, pet danders, dust, and smoke, and destroys viruses, bacteria, mold and mildews.

For More Information

Airwise air purifiers: Visit www.RenewYourself.net and click appliances. Click the Contact button and email me for your special discount coupon code.

PART 5: HEALTHY THERAPIES AND PRACTICES

Chiropractic

At the age of 18 I fell asleep at the wheel of my VW Bug and ran into a telephone pole at 60 mph. The trauma to my neck and body was quite significant. I sought the help of a chiropractor and had an amazing, life-altering experience. Because of that experience, I felt called into chiropractic practice where I have been for over 25 years. I have also personally experienced the work of more than 75 chiropractors.

It is my hope to dispel some common myths and misunderstandings about chiropractic, and to address some well-founded apprehensions and concerns about it. The benefits of chiropractic when done correctly can be truly remarkable.

Manual Manipulation

Many people are terrified of having their necks manually adjusted, i.e., "cracking the neck." The problem seems to be that many practitioners apply non-specific adjustments to the neck, with high rotational force. In other words, they twist the neck with their adjustments. This can present several problems.

First, if the doctor has not isolated specific segments that are hypo-mobile (have restricted motion), he or she can create hypermobility or laxity (looseness) in areas of the spine that are already moving properly. This can be irritating to the ligaments and other soft tissue structures. If the patient tenses his muscles in anticipation of this, it can compound the problems.

Second, when vertebral joints in the neck are manipulated using high-velocity rotational components, the stretch reflex is often initiated, causing the muscles to contract in the local area as a protective mechanism. This often results in the vertebrae subluxating (dislocating) or mal-positioning worse than before the attempted correction.

Research at the Pettibon Institute, by Dr. Burl Pettibon, has demonstrated through video fluoroscopy or movie x-rays that manual adjustments of this type to the cervical spine indeed make the patient's condition worse over time, often producing pathology. Adjusting other areas of the spine that are compensatory in nature may further compound the problems.

So what is the solution?

1. Your doctor should "motion palpate" the segments of the cervical spine (feel each spinal joint as it moves through its range of motion), looking for areas of restricted motion.

2. If the doctor uses manual manipulation, he or she should not apply rotational forces to the neck! While he or she may put the neck in a slight rotational position before initiating the adjustment, he or she should not apply rotational force. The chin should not twist or move in a torquing manner.

3. While some initial tenderness may occur during the first several visits, it should not be severe. Rather, a tenderness something like that of working out at a gym for the first time after a several-month hiatus is acceptable for the first several visits. Extreme pain or prolonged tenderness is not acceptable.

4. If the doctor manually manipulates the cervical spine, there should be no twisting. The force applied should instead be more of an axial decompression type.

5. The doctor may apply instrument adjusting or reflex-type work as an alternative to manual manipulation.

6. The doctor should periodically monitor your response to care by re-evaluating your range of motion. In other words, you should experience an increased ability to move your neck and spine through different planes of movement. A baseline evaluation of your condition should be taken, using surface electromyographic (sEMG) examination. sEMG scanning is a painless way to make the electrical activity of your nervous system visible. Your doctor should be experienced and skilled at performing this test, and the equipment must be calibrated

correctly. Your scans should show visible improvement at periodic intervals.

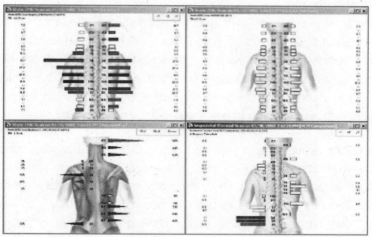

SEMG results showing electrical activity surrounding spine

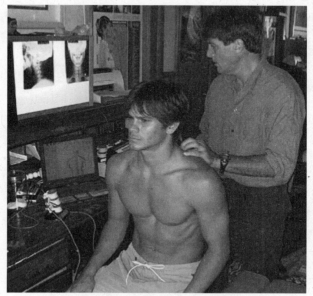

Dr. Cromack performing SEMG scan on Myles Padaca

ArthroStim

An alternative to manual adjusting is the ArthroStim, a safe and effective electromechanical adjusting instrument that gently taps the vertebrae back into place. The ArthroStim works is particularly useful for pain-sensitive or older individuals. It generates 15 impulses of energy per second, which allow the neural receptors to quickly relay information to the brain. The clinician can modulate the depth and force of the adjusting heads from very light to extremely deep and also to choose the direction of the drive.

ArthroStim delivers input into the nervous system by generating 12-14 incremental thrusts per second. With the reception of these rapid impulses, your neural receptors are able to then quickly relay this crucial information to the brain. The brain proceeds to use this neurological feedback to issue self-correcting commands to bring about the healing aid needed in the muscular systems. I have never heard a patient say that they did not enjoy the feeling of being adjusted with the ArthroStim and have found it to be a useful alternative or adjunct to traditional manual adjustment techniques.

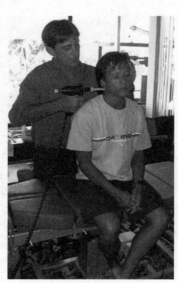

ArthroStim adjustment

Choosing a Chiropractor

Be wary of any chiropractor who uses big practice-management schemes and tries to sell you a lengthy prepaid treatment plan. An initial trial of 10 to 12 visits is appropriate, and you should experience relief by the fourth to sixth visit.

Look for a doctor who is experienced and who can readily provide multiple good referrals. He or she should know how to make use of drop tables, and the newer electronic adjusting instruments. If a patient is over 50, or is apprehensive of manual manipulation, the chiropractor should rely more on instrument adjusting and non-force techniques, as opposed to manual adjusting.

Look for someone with a background in acupuncture, herbology, detoxification methods, live food nutrition, and exercise. Look for someone who has great hands and can adjust manually and smoothly if needed. And perhaps most important, look for a doctor who has a big heart, walks his or her talk, and inspires you.

Your chiropractor should encourage and motivate you to take responsibility for your well-being, emphasizing lifestyle practices, such as diet, exercise, relaxation, supplementation, and the like, which act synergistically to improve quality of life and health. If he or she instead makes endless recommendations of frequent adjustments, you need to find another doctor.

Chiropractic is an art, and although the training and qualifications are intense and some incredible doctors are out there, not everyone is going to be a great chiropractor. Some people have a strong intellect, but not great hands. Others excel great academically and have a big heart, but can't put it all together.

What makes a great musician, surgeon, or artist? Some are born with the "touch." Others grow into it, and still others will never mature into greatness. Of the seventy-five chiropractors that I have seen, some were not good, some were okay, and then there were the ten who really helped me.

Chiropractic Benefits

Your spine is how life travels through your body—from your brain down the spinal cord, via the spinal nerve trunks, to every cell, tissue, and organ of your body. If you are getting appropriate chiropractic care, you will experience positive changes to your central nervous system over time, such as the following:

- Increased synchronization of the right and left hemispheres of your brain.
- Increased endorphin production.
- Increased cerebrospinal fluid pressure.
- Increased alpha brain wave patterns, and decreased beta brain wave patterns during activity, indicating enhanced relaxation.
- Decreased pain, better sleep, more mental clarity, energy, and overall well-being.

If you have not had a great chiropractic experience in the past, I understand. I encourage you to remain open minded and pray to be guided to those who will help you. The word *doctor* means teacher. When the student is ready, the teacher will appear. It takes time and patience to heal.

Chiropractic applied properly, by the right hands, works in concert with the other recommendations in this book to produce superb health.

Acupuncture

Acupuncture is the ancient art of balancing the meridians or energy pathways along which life force or qi (pronounced "chi") moves thru our bodies. By stimulating certain points along the twelve meridians on each side of your body, we can balance the meridians, and facilitate healing. We can stimulate these points by needles, lasers, electricity, or physical pressure (acupressure). Stimulating a point along a meridian influences either the organ associated with the meridian or the area that the meridian traverses.

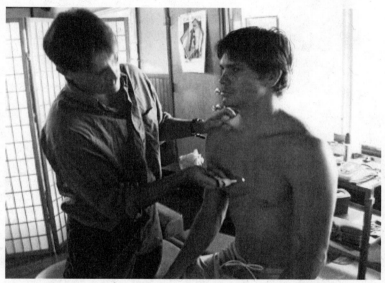

Dr. Cromack using laser to stimulate the conception vessel.

Electro Meridian Imaging (EMI) graphs a visual analysis of the twelve meridians on both sides of the body. From this information, we can see which meridians need to be balanced and zero in the most effective treatment plan.

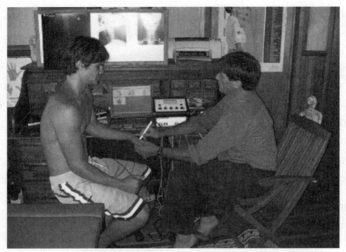

Myles Padaca receiving electromeridian imaging

Electromeridian Imaging

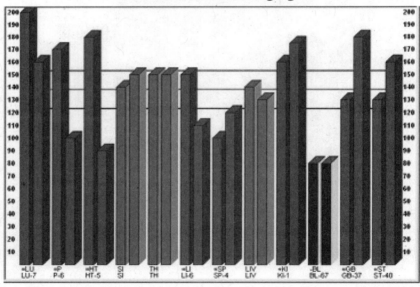

Graph of all 12 EMI meridians on the right and left side of the body

Pictorial Acupressure Guide

This pictorial series will teach you how to stimulate acupuncture points for treatment of low back pain, elbow, shoulder, and wrist pain, as well as headaches and insomnia. Do not attempt if pregnant.

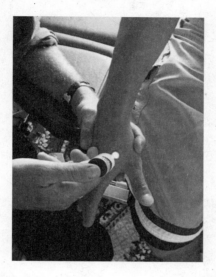

The HoKu Master point for arm pain located in the middle of the thumb web. Helps wrist, elbow, shoulder, neck pain, and headaches. Dr. Cromack is using special frequency laser.

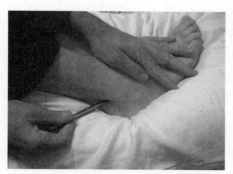

The Kun Lun point is located on both legs, in the groove formed between the Achilles tendon and the outside ankle bone and helps with back pain, sciatica, leg and buttock pain.

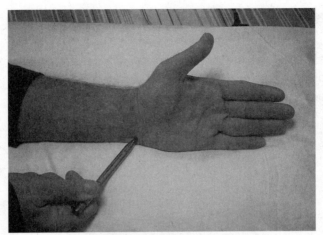

The Shen Men point, located on the wrist crease, on the inside of the tendon at the lateral edge of the wrist, is helpful for quieting the spirit, insomnia, and nervousness.

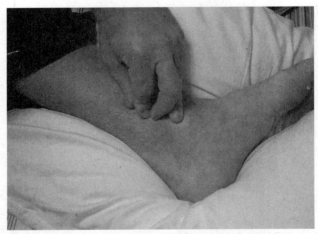

The Three Mile Spleen 6 point is located four fingers or 3 human inches above the center of the medial maleolus, just on the back side of the tibia where you will feel a slight indentation behind the Tibia. Spleen 6 is good for sickness and menstrual cramps. Massage the appropriate point on each side of body for 3-5 minutes.

Renew Yourself!

Youthing and Regeneration Program

The Renew Yourself! Rejuvenation and Youthing program was formulated by Dr. Gabriel Cousens, M.D., and myself. The program combines over 65 years of clinical experience. A neuro-diagnostic computer scan measures the electrical activity emanating from the spine, from the upper cervical area to the sacrum. The visual results then form a baseline for each patient. Combined with a physical examination and medical history, the physician creates an individualized approach to achieve optimal health.

The Renew Yourself! program understands that the central nervous system is how life travels through your body. Messages start in your brain and travel down your spinal cord via your spinal nerve roots; to every cell, tissue, organ, gland, and muscle in your body. If you can remove obstruction to this communication pathway, life is expressed more clearly. Your body is self healing and self regulating. When you provide your body with clean food, air, water, rest, exercise, sunshine and positive thoughts, your body has the best chance of healing itself.

The Renew Yourself program addresses a new paradigm in health. Traditional health care is a sickness model concerned with relieving pain and symptoms. It assumes that health is the absence of disease or symptoms. The Renew Yourself program is interested in giving the experience of the increasing levels of Wellness that lie between no symptoms and optimum functioning of the nervous system or full-body enlightenment.

The Tree of Life Rejuvenation Center has incorporated this powerful treatment into its world-renowned 10-day, 17-day and 24-day detoxification retreats, Reversing Diabetes, cancer prevention, and mental wellness programs, as well as its spiritual juice fasting retreats. The effects, when combined with juice fasting, speed the process of breaking down adhesions and calcifications. When combined with supplementation from the *Longevity*

Now Program developed by David Wolfe, the synergistic effect dramatically activates anti-aging, anti-inflammatory, anti-cancer and antioxidant genes.

Techniques used in the Renew Yourself! Program, verified by University of Texas research, create an increased synchronization of the left and right hemisphere of the brain, increased endorphin release, and enable a more relaxed Alpha brain wave pattern. Since the inception of the program the results have been consistent: Over 95% of the patients report an increase in clarity and sense of well-being, ranging from a mild contentment to heightened states of euphoria. Often there is a dramatic release of unresolved emotional trauma that gets locked in the soft tissue and the spinal cord. With the release of these blockages, there is usually a catharsis, or purification of unresolved emotions on a spiritual level. As the patient releases repressed emotions the nervous system is restored to its optimum state.

Patients also experience a dramatic increase in energy, clarity and well-being, and many of the middle aged and older patients report increased range of motion, most notably in the cervical spine. We have had a number of patients in their fifties and sixties come in with a 25 to 50% reduction of their ability to rotate their head due to stiffness. Three weeks later, many leave with 70 to 95% of the normal range of motion of a twenty-five year old person. From a medical perspective, these results are quite dramatic.

The Tree of Life teaches guests many different lifestyle tools that can be used at home to continue the process of growing, expansion, and healing. Experience organic nutrient-dense vegetable juices and gourmet live-food, mediation, clean air, nature walks, yoga, and many other medical and spa services. Many seeds are planted here for the journey of living a truly liberated life.

For More Information

To learn more about Renew Yourself! and the Tree of Life Rejuvenation Center, visit www.TreeofLife.nu/renewyourself.

Restorative Stretching

These poses use your own bodyweight over blankets and bolsters to stretch over-contracted soft tissue and help to achieve balance. They also help to reduce the effect of stress-related disease. When your mind and body perceive something as life threatening, the physiological response is of a stressful nature. The adrenal glands react by secreting adrenaline and noradrenalin; which act upon the autonomic nervous system to prepare us for fight or flight. Digestion, elimination, growth, and repair slow down. Blood pressure, heart rate, mental alertness, and muscle tension increase. Modern man spends too much time in this mode and doesn't know how to break the cycle.

The solution to stress is deep relaxation and rest. By focusing the mind on the breath with the eyes closed, while doing the restorative poses, a deep state of relaxation is achieved. The rest achieved by doing this can be much deeper than many parts of the sleep cycle.

The poses are designed to move the spine in all directions. It is important to get forward bending, back bending, twisting, and side bending poses into your daily routine. An inverted pose tones the heart by allowing fluid that has accumulated in the legs from sitting and standing, to return to the upper body.

The poses also provide a squeezing and massaging effect to the internal organs, which helps move out stagnant blood and bring in fresh blood, oxygen and nutrients. This has a tonifying effect. Try to do the poses daily. Hold each pose for 30 seconds. If this is comfortable, gradually extend each pose up to 3-4 minutes or longer. Make sure your rib cage lifts away from the internal organs with each inhalation, and with each exhalation let your belly soften and your mind quiet. Keep your awareness on your breath and the area between your eyebrows.

For More Information

Buy your copy of the amazing book *Relax & Renew: Restful Yoga for Stressful* Times by Judith Lasater at www.RenewYourself.net.

Elevated Legs Up the Wall Pose

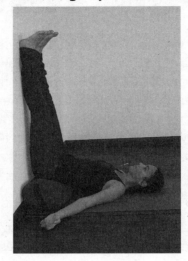

Supported Forward Bend

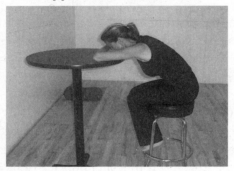

Simple Forward Bends For Home Or Office

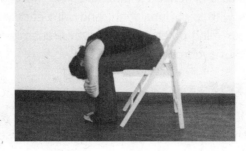

Simple Supported Back Bend

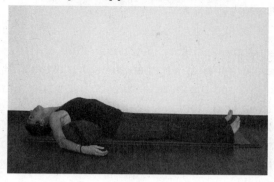

Supported Spinal Twist

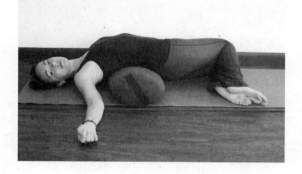

Supported Bound Angle Pose

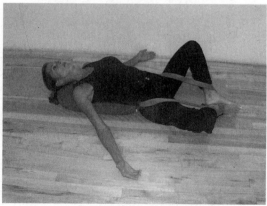

Scoliosis

Scoliosis is a frequently hereditary lateral curvature of the spine. In working with scoliosis we are trying to lengthen the spine overall. At the same time we are trying to balance the musculature of the spine by stretching over-contracted muscles and toning weak musculature. A combination of restorative stretches, decompression, lengthening with an inversion sling, and swimming are complementary to possible appropriate chiropractic care in de-rotating the spine and rib cage. You should be doing the following restorative poses daily.

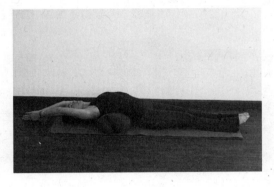

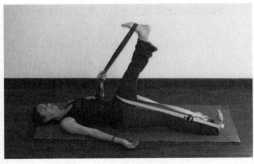

Note: Before doing this pose stand in front of a mirror and put your hands on the sides of the pelvic bone, to decide which hip is higher. The purple strap needs to go over the top of the thigh on the side that is higher.

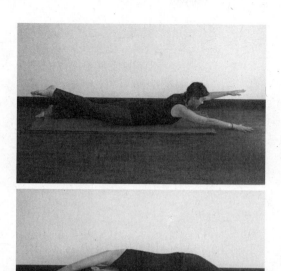

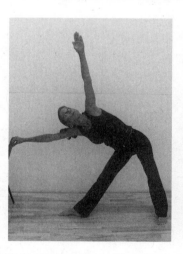

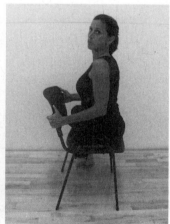

For More Information

Buy *Yoga for Scoliosis* by Elise B. Miller at www.RenewYourself.net.

Rehabilitative Stretching

If you have any pain, injury or stiffness in your body, you should review the stretching programs prepared by Mary Hutto, MS,RPT,LMT of Maui. She organized these safe effective stretches that she has used in her physical therapy practice for over 18 years, that have given her patients lasting relief. These unique stretches give break through results and are presented in animation form to that you can easily see and understand how to perform each stretch correctly. The stretches target specific muscles that are causing the pain, limitation in mobility and poor posture.

She has DVDS for each 10 joint areas. specialty DVDs and DVDS for common sports. The DVDs are available thru http://www.RenewYourself.net.

Stretching is one of the most important things you can do to keep you injury and pain free as well as prevent a lot of unnecessary degeneration to your body. Since muscles cross over the joints they move, when they tighten they compress the joint that they cross. Long term compression leads to tendonitis, bursitis and eventually osteoarthritis.

Many injuries end up with fibrin or scar tissue, in and around the area of involvement. Fibrin is a cheaper grade of tissue than normal soft tissue, has less elasticity than healthy tissue, and can be up to seventy times more pain sensitive than normal tissue. Doing the proper rehabilitative stretches at the appropriate time, helps minimize the over production of scar tissue, helps increase circulation to decrease pain and spasm and helps one to regain and maintain normal range of motion. The DVDS are animated and are full of not widely known information. They are the next best thing to having a Physical Therapist with you.

For More Information

Visit www.RenewYourself.net and click on Neck and Back Health for Mary Smithson-Hutto DVDs and more.

Strength Training

It is essential to develop a strength training program for yourself. Hormones begin to shift after thirty. Growth hormone begins to decrease in both men and women by the early thirties. Testosterone levels also decline in men. Women also experience a shift of hormones during menopause making them more susceptible to osteoporosis. These hormone shifts make it more difficult to maintain lean muscle mass and strength as we get older, and contribute to an increase in inter-abdominal fat.

A study by the AMA reported a 48 percent increase in mobility and huge increases of strength in a group of ten ninety year olds that trained for eight weeks. Cardio exercise such as Brisk walking, swimming, or cycling meets of at least 30 minutes four to five times a week is also essential for health.

One of the more amazing examples I have seen of the role of strength training and nutrition in longevity is Dr. Bob Delmontique. Dr. Delmontique looks better physique wise at 84 than at 19 while training for the football team. Check out his website at bobdelmontique.com.

A study done at Harvard University on the 17,000 male alumni compared the participants' average calories per week of exercise to their longevity:

- Those who did about 500 calories per week in exercise had the highest death rate.

- Those doing 500-1000 calories of exercise per week saw a 22% reduction in mortality.

- Those doing 3500 calories, or about 5-10 hours per week had a 54% improvement in longevity.

- Those doing more than 10 hours a week of exercise dropped down to a 38% improvement in longevity.

It should be obvious that more in not necessarily better. Too much exercise increases cortisol and decreases DHEA. Over training increases free radical production, and weakens the immune system. The proper amount increases testosterone, immune system function, and increases muscle mass, while decreasing cortisol.

It takes about 30-45 minutes of cardio to reach the **Tranquillizer Effect.** There is up to a 500% increase in endorphins that are more powerful than morphine. The effect lasts about 5 hours.

The optimum pulse rate is about 180 minus the person's age. The optimal amount of training will vary from person to person depending on body type, and age. The minimum is about 35 minutes of cardio daily and strength training twice a week with one to two sets of resistance for each body part. After 45 minutes of strength training testosterone levels drop by 90 Percent. Additional work after this point is counterproductive.

It is important to put an easy to digest nutrient dense drink in the first 30 minutes after finishing training. My super smoothie is great, and if you are going to the gym, taking a thermos of it with you for afterwards is a good idea. Avoid sweets and starches that raise your blood sugar levels rapidly afterwards, it will sabotage much of the good work you have done.

Getting enough rest after strength training and exercise is just as important as the exercise. Some professional athletes are experimenting with using mind machines (Holosync sound technology) after training to produce states of delta brain wave patterns which increase the secretion of HGH or Human Growth Hormone. Make sure you have your super smoothie first.

It is my opinion much of your remaining training time should be filled out with restorative stretches as well as breathing exercise, and relaxation techniques. This will provide a nice balance.

For More Information

Click on Peter Ragnar at www.renewyourself.net for your copy of his amazing book, *Serious Strength:For Seniors and Kids under 65.*

Breathing Exercises

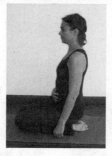

Relax the diaphragm and fill the lower lung. Move the air up into the upper lung. Then reverse the sequence ending by contracting the diaphragm and expelling as much old air as possible.

Deep breathing is a way to super oxygenate our blood stream, and fill our body with Prana or Life Force. The average person exchanges about a pint of air on each inhalation and exhalation. The lung capacity is about 7-10 pints. You can get about 7 times more oxygen and Prana by doing deep breathing. This super charging brings extra life and connects the mind and breath. Deep breathing slows the mind. As the mind slows, breath becomes smoother.

Deep breathing has a very calming effect on the mind and nervous system. It balances the sympathetic and parasympathetic nervous systems. Regular practice of deep breathing with right living brings purification of the nadis or subtle nerve channels. As the nadis become purified, the body starts to become very light (culminating in a sense of weightlessness) The eyes become brighter, digestion sounder, sleep better, and skin more radiant. These are signs associated with radiant health!

As bodily functions improve and the body purifies many of the aches, pains, and stiffness you have will begin to disappear. Deep breathing should relax the diaphragm on inhalation filling the lungs from bottom to top. Exhalation should use the diaphragm at the end to squeeze out as much old air as possible.

Alternate Nostril Breathing

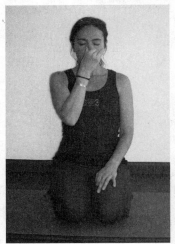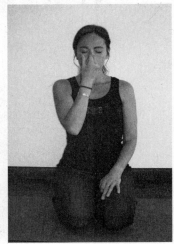

Close the right nostril with the right thumb, exhale air completely out of the left. Continue holding the right nostril closed and inhale a slow deep breath thru the left nostril, when your lungs have taken as much air in as possible, close the left nostril with the right 4th and 5th finger. Then exhale the air out thru the right nostril. Upon emptying the right nostril, inhale thru the right nostril, then close the right nostril with the right thumb and exhale thru the left nostril. This completes one round. You would then continue by again inhaling thru the left nostril and continue with the cycle described above.

It is important to develop a smoothness and rhythm to the breathing. The breathing should not be jerky or hurried. Keep the awareness on the breath and the point between the eyes, eventually a rhythm of twice as long for exhalation as inhalation will develop.

Do not practice for 3 hours after a full meal. One hour after a light snack is OK. Start with 10 rounds a day at one sitting.

Meditation

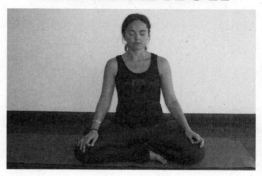

We don't need to over mystify meditation. To keep it simple, think of praying as talking to God, and meditating as listening to what he has to say. A daily meditation program is indispensable in healing and achieving optimal health. Start with a short regular practice of say 10 minutes a day, something you can easily accomplish on a regular basis. This allows us time to get into the habit of making a space in our day to be quiet and still. It allows us to develop a short practice that we look forward to.

It is important to sit with the back straight. For most people this is easier with a pillow under the buttocks to rock the pelvis forward, as well as a small pillow supporting the lumbar curve. Alternatively, kneeling with a pillow between the legs is comfortable for others. Start by closing your eyes and putting your awareness between the eyebrows. Feel your breath coming in and out. On the in breath repeat "I" and on the out breath repeat "AM".

With regular practice the mind becomes one pointed, and the breath and metabolic rate slow down considerably allowing for deep relaxation and rest. The brain wave patterns shift from a beta pattern to more of an alpha brain wave pattern consistent with deep relaxation. There is an increased synchronization of the two hemispheres of the brain and healing is accelerated. Over time you can gradually increase the length of practice. A shorter regular practice is much better than sporadically for longer periods of time.

Fasting

"Anything can be achieved in small, deliberate steps. But there are times you need the courage to take a great leap. You can't cross a chasm in two small jumps" - David Lloyd George

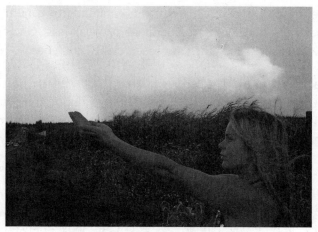

Photo courtesy of Scott Perez

Fasting holds amazing possibilities for rejuvenation and healing. Some fasters have even reported psychic experiences during long fasts. Dormant higher spiritual centers can become active as a result of fasting.

Fasting activates the youthing genes. Reducing the intake of calories has repetitively shown to have a life extension effect. The best way to achieve a youthing and life extension effect is through eating an easy-to-digest, nutrient-dense, live food diet which allows us to satisfy our nutritional needs with much smaller quantities of food, and periodic juice fasts.

Water fasting should only be attempted by experienced fasters. Fasting with a majority of fresh squeezed green vegetable juices and E3Live® (see page 37), mixed with a little fresh squeezed apple juice is ideal. The trick is to allow for plenty of alkalizing minerals from the greens, which help to buffer the toxins coming out, and to minimize higher glycemic fruit juices.

Juice fasting allows us to divert energy normally used for digestion into detoxifying non vital tissue. The body will detoxify accumulated toxins from the most recent backwards towards birth. When the body goes through an accelerated cleansing the toxins come out through the organs of elimination. This means that during cleansing palpitations, pimples, bad breath, headaches, nausea, runs, sweats, and itching are all possible at different times. These symptoms can last from a few minutes to a number of days. These episodes often include an experience of weakness. Once the episode passes you will usually experience increased clarity and energy.

The healthier you are the longer you can fast and the less discomfort you feel. You will probably only experience hunger during the first three days of juice fasting. If your body is cleansed, by the fourth day a feeling of euphoria, lightness and energy usually supersedes the temporary abstinence of food.

If you have chronic pain, stiffness, and discomfort in your body, each 7-10 day juice fast you do will lessen your pain and stiffness and improve your energy, clarity, and overall appearance. If you are inexperienced in fasting, I recommend that you do this under the supervision of a licensed health practitioner experienced in this area. You should not fast if you have diabetes, certain cancers, or are considerably underweight or debilitated. Always check with your doctor first, especially if you are taking medications. Do not attempt a 7-10 day juice fast initially if you have been eating a lot of processed junk food, meat, and dairy. Do not undertake a fast when you are under extreme pressure or working full time.

I recommend that most people first do several one day and three day juice fasts, before proceeding to a 7-10 day juice fast. After a fast, your taste is resensitised, and eliminating less desirable food is easier.

Instructions:
- The day before the fast, just have a fresh made vegetable soup or juicy fruit for dinner, and fruit or smoothie for lunch. Have some herb tea in the evening and take a solid dose of about 8 Triphala.

- Do not drink straight fruit juice. You can drink up to four 20 oz. fresh squeezed vegetable drinks. I recommend celery, cucumber, kale, apple, with a pinch of lemon juice. The juice should be about 1/3 apple juice. The drink should be mixed with one tablespoon of E3Live® (see page 37).
- Avoid over-exertion, excessive sun, or drafts. A light swim or walk is good. Avoid swimming in chlorinated water.
- Practice restorative stretches, meditating, and deep breathing.
- Do dry skin massage with a brush.
- Take at least one enema daily to flush the lower GI tract. Do not use tap water.
- Allow plenty of rest and quiet. Fill the mind with spiritually uplifting thoughts.
- Take 2 enzyme capsules every 2 hours.
- Take probiotics for one week after finishing the fast, to re-establish normal GI flora.

Fasting and Detoxification with E3Live

The standard American diet requires great amounts of physical energy to digest and eliminate. Assimilation is usually poor, and toxins are often generated as by-products. These toxins lodge in the cells, intracellular fluids, colon, joints, and muscles. They clog the microcirculatory energy channels in our bodies and contribute to stiffness, aging, loss of energy, and reduced well-being. It is not unusual to experience some periods of detoxification when fasting or taking larger doses of E3Live®. When you juice fast with E3Live®, you divert some of the energy that your body would normally use for digestion into internal house cleaning and detoxification. Symptoms may be experienced as the toxins flow into the bloodstream and pass through the various organs of elimination. They may include headaches, nausea, loose stools, itching, pimples, foul breath, weakness, heart palpations, and sweats. These can last from hours to a few days if you follow the above recommendations. This is followed by an increase in well-being and health. Take naps and get extra rest as your body goes through these healing crises.

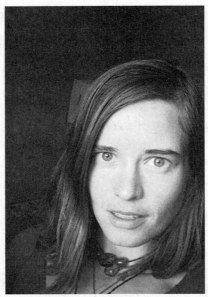

Angela Stokes at the end of her 92 day "juice feast"

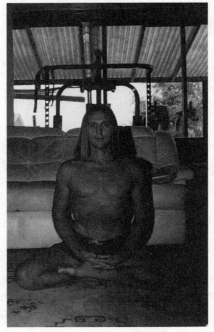

The author at age 43 on day 72 of a E3Live® Aquabotanical juice fast

Essential Renewal Practices

In this section I briefly outline additional highly beneficial practices for your physical, mental, and spiritual health. As with the rest of the book, my experience with the benefits of these practices is first hand both through my personal practice and through witnessing the transformation of my patients.

Home Rejuvenation Therapy

While the experience of an in residence rejuvenation program lead to profound well-being and joy, the cost can sometimes be prohibitive. I am going to give you instruction for doing a home rejuvenation treatment on yourself. While not as profound as a professional retreat, the results are often great. I suggest a 5 day home treatment program. Do not attempt a prolonged program at home. This treatment can be a little messy at home and does take a little time; having said that, it is doable and fairly inexpensive. I strongly recommend this program. You will feel much lighter, and more alive!

Instructions: Therapy starts with internal oilation. Traditionally this is done with ghee, but raw coconut oil can be substituted for the ghee. For 4 mornings in a row you are going to take increasing amounts of oil on an empty stomach; starting with 2 teaspoons the first morning, 4 the next and 6 on the third and fourth morning. I suggest buying some chai flavoured almond milk and warming about 6 oz. of the chai almond milk and melting the dose of ghee or coconut oil into it. On the 4th evening take a hot bath for about 20 minutes. Take 4 Triphala before going to bed. On the morning of the 5ᵗʰ day, mix 4 oz. castor oil into ½ cup of fresh-squeezed grapefruit juice, hold your nose and chug. Bite into an orange afterwards. Be at home for the next 5 hours! You need to be off work this day.

You should be on an ama-reducing diet during this home treatment. It's best to eat blended warm veggie soups and light, easy to digest food.

External oilation begins the day after the castor oil purgative. You will do extended abhyanga as described in the manual. You are going to sit on a large towel, with 6 oz. of warm sesame oil. You are going to spend 20 minutes rubbing your body thoroughly from head to toe with the warm oil. Then you are going to prepare a hot bath and soak for 20 minutes.

You should be taking 6-8 Triphala capsules every night before going to bed and drinking at least 6 cups of warm distilled water a day.

On day 2 and 4 of the external oilation and following the hot bath, you are going to purge the lower colon with about a 16 oz. Clear water basti (enema). You are going to evacuate, then follow this with a mildly warm 8 oz. sesame oil basti which you will try to retain for 10 minutes.

The positive results of the 5 day rejuvenation therapy will be more evident about a week following the program.

Holosync

The Holosync audio technology uses binaural beats to produce alpha, theta, and delta states. The listener sits quietly with eyes closed and listens to relaxing environmental sounds on headphones. I find it relaxing to do while meditating on the breath.

It often takes Zen monks 20 years of daily practice consisting of hours of daily meditation, before they can quickly produce theta brain wave patterns. The Holosync audio program allows practitioners to quickly duplicate the same brain wave patterns as experienced Zen meditators.

There is increased synchronization of two hemispheres of the brain, which indicates more harmonious functioning.

Because of the deep relaxation associated with the alpha, theta, and delta states, stress hormones like cortisol are reduced. Healthy hormones like DHEA, melatonin, and HGH increase. Endorphins that make us feel that natural high are increased.

Sun Gazing

Gazing at the setting sun a **half hour** before sunset has a harmonizing effect upon nervous system and the endocrine glands, particularly the pineal gland. Start with 10 seconds, one half hour before sunset. The tangential plane of the sun in the last half hour before it sets makes this practice safe. With consistent practice, you can add 10 seconds every other day, working up to 10 minutes. This improves both the immune system and depression.

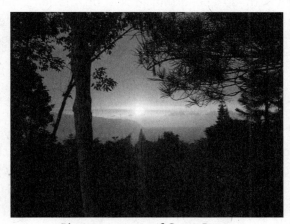

Photo courtesy of Scott Perez

Papaya Enzyme Facial

The effects of this facial, done weekly, are immediate and cumulative.

- Apply mashed papaya enzyme mask for 10 minutes and rinse
- Boil water with one teaspoon of chopped ginger in it for 10 minutes. Turn it off and drape a towel over your head and the pot, for about 5 to 10 minutes. Be careful not to burn yourself!
- Massage lightly with E3Live® (see page 37). Lightly polish to exfoliate dead skin and toxins, rinse.
- Apply clay mask for 15 minutes to draw out toxins and tighten skin.
- Rinse and apply mask of Monuka honey for 15 minutes.
- Rinse and apply E3Live® light crème and leave.

Abhyanga Oil Massage

Abhyanga is an external oilation massage treatment. Abhyanga can be done daily or weekly. It has a rejuvenating effect on the physiology, and is extremely purifying to the nervous system. I recommend using the best quality sesame oil. In a tropical environment during summer, coconut oil is cooling.

Instructions: Sit on a towel. Warm the oil to about 110 degrees. Massage the oil with up and down strokes on the long bones, and in a circular motion over the elbows, knees, shoulders, scalp, and feet. Let the oil absorb for 10 minutes then take a long hot shower. Abhyanga rejuvenates by promoting the ojas (subtle nerve force).

Ejuva

If you want to make a dramatic change quickly in the way you think, feel, and look, I strongly recommend that you must try the Ejuva cleanse. These images are actual photos of what comes out of the colon during an Ejuva cleanse. The late Dr. John Kellogg performed more than 10,000 autopsies and declared not one person had a normal colon.

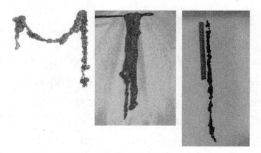

Photo courtesy of www.ejuva.com

Most people have up to a half inch thick of encrusted mucoid plaque in the 30 feet of GI tubing that comprises their large and small intestine. This radically interferes with absorption of nutrients, as well as creating a condition of auto-intoxication of our blood stream. The Ejuva cleanse is a 30 day program of a hand prepared blend of herbs that have a softening effect on this plaque, allowing us to eliminate it. After eliminating the mucoid plaque, the experience is one of increased clarity, well-being, and energy. You may need to do up to 8 of these cleanses at 6 month intervals while eating a cleansing diet, to eliminate all the stubborn plaque. I recommend waiting to do an Ejuva cleanse until you have been taking E3Live® (see page 37) for at least 5 months and are eating a healthy, natural diet. Then you will be ready to experience the amazing regenerative power of an Ejuva cleanse.

For More Information

Visit www.renewyourself.net and click on Ejuva Cleanse.

Implants

A useful tool during cleansing, detox, and fasting can be the implant. After clearing the lower colon with a basti (water enema), another smaller basti of about 4-6 ounces of wheatgrass juice or E3Live® (see page 37) is administered. It should be retained for about 10 minutes. Pressing on the perineum (the area between the genitals and anus) will help get one thru the first several minutes when an urge to evacuate may come with some contractile spasms. The chlorophyll is absorbed through the lower GI tract and it often has the effect of clearing cloudiness in the head.

Tongue Scraping

Tongue scraping is one of the Shat-Karmas (physical cleansings) that help us rid our bodies of excessive mucus and toxins. They smooth and speed recovery from initial cleansing symptoms and can result in an immediate shift in your experience. You will often feel much lighter afterwards.

All of us should use a tongue scraper in the morning in addition to brushing and flossing the teeth and gargling with salt water. Tongue scraping is part of normal hygiene. During periods of fasting and cleansing, the tongue can become heavily coated.

Stomach Washing

This practice cleanses acids, bile, and undigested ferments from the stomach. If you feel nauseous or experience undigested food from the day before, the stomach wash can be a useful tool, especially to relieve detox. The stomach wash is not to be confused with bulimia. It should be done only one morning per week, on an empty stomach and not during winter months.

Instructions: Mix 2 teaspoons of Himalayan Crystal Salt with one liter of tepid purified water. Drink 10 gulps at a time, finishing the litre over a 3-5 minute period. Bend forward over the toilet and stimulate the gag reflex, by holding the finger or a tooth brush against the uvula, until the water is regurgitated. You may have to repeat this a few times to get most of the saline rinse out. Usually a decrease in stomach discomfort and headache is experienced, followed by a significant increase in mental clarity.

Sinus Wash

The sinus wash helps relieve the build up of congestion in sinus problems and head colds and washes out excess phlegm.

Instructions: Mix one teaspoon of Himalayan Crystal Salt with a pint of purified tepid water in a large bowl. Stick your nose in it over the bathroom sink. Pull up slowly and steadily until the water comes down the back of the throat. Without swallowing the rinse, spit out and repeat.

Dry Skin Brushing

The skin is the largest organ of the body. Since your skin is one of the organs of elimination, dry skin brushing is a tool which can speed up your detoxification. By taking a dry skin brush and brushing your skin all over your body for 5 minutes daily you will slough off the old dead skin and increase blood flow to the surface of the skin. You will notice a mist of dead skin in the air as you do it.

Epilogue

Now you have finished the book. If most of this material is new to you, you might feel overwhelmed, or not know where to start. Please remember that you don't need to integrate everything in this book all at once. If you need help figuring out where to start there are many resources available on my website, www.RenewYourself.net. I am also available for phone consultation.

May God guide you on your journey.

George Cromack, D.C., F.I.A.M.A.

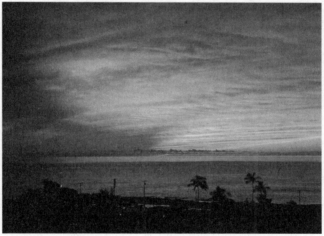

Photo: Ron Condon

"Nothing real can be threatened. Nothing unreal exists. Therein lies the peace of God." - A Course in Miracles